THE ULTIMATE CANDIDA GUIDE

AND COOKBOOK©

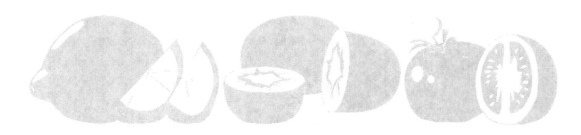

The Breakthrough Plan for Eliminating Disease Causing Yeast

and Revolutionizing Your Health!

Including over 150 Candida Fighting Recipes

BY DR COBI SLATER, PHD, DNM®, RHT, RNCP

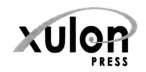

PRESS

The Ultimate Candida Guide and Cookbook
The Breakthrough Plan for Eliminating Disease Causing Yeast and Revolutionizing Your Health!
by Dr Cobi Slater, PhD, DNM®, RHT, RNCP

Printed in the United States of America

ISBN 9781629520209

This book is not intended as a substitute for the medical advice of physicians. The reader should regularly consult a physician in matters relating to his/her health and particularly with respect to any symptoms that may require diagnosis or medical attention.

www.xulonpress.com

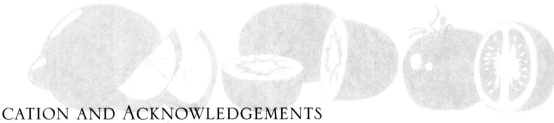

DEDICATION AND ACKNOWLEDGEMENTS

This book is dedicated to the many patients who poured their hearts out and entrusted the hope of a healthier future with me. I witnessed each of you boldly embrace enough courage to carve a new path for yourselves with a life free from the symptoms that plagued you. I am honored to be a part of your healing journey.

I wish to especially thank my Mom, Arlene Kubin who sat with me by the hour to finish this book. Mom, you are my inspiration and without your guidance, I would be lost. I would also like to thank my husband Garry who fearlessly allows me to embrace each new dream. To my boys, Dane and Kade, you are my world and I cherish every moment with you. Thank you to my Dad, who continually supports me, talks with me by the hour and gives my Mom the freedom to do all she does for me.

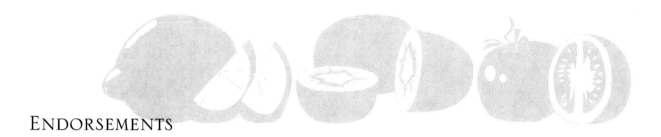

ENDORSEMENTS

" D r. Cobi Slater is one of the brightest health professionals I've had the privilege of knowing. If you are suffering from a candida infection (and most people are), I encourage you to read her book "The Ultimate Candida Guide and Cookbook". It is the definitive guide on the subject and a manual to restore your health. Packed with important information and recipes, everyone should read this book and apply the wisdom within its pages."

Michelle Schoffro Cook, MS, PhD, RNCP, ROHP, DNM

International best-selling author of *60 Seconds to Slim*, *Weekend Wonder Detox*, and *The Ultimate pH Solution*. DrMichelleCook.com

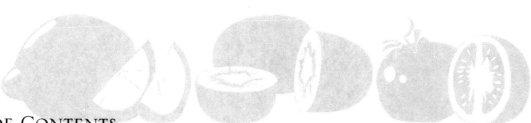

TABLE OF CONTENTS

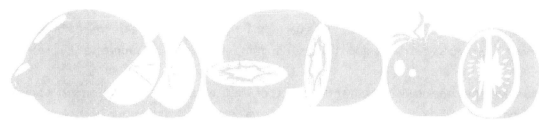

INTRODUCTION TO CANDIDA

C andida albicans is a specific fungus or form of yeast found living in the intestinal tracts of most individuals. Candida can be an invasive problem that can drain energy stores, disrupt digestive function, deplete the immune system and cause the liver to be stressed as well as interrupt hormone balance and result in mood swings. People with Candida often suffer from the following common symptoms:

COMMON SYMPTOMS OF CANDIDA
- **General**: chronic fatigue, sweet cravings, weight gain, skin conditions (acne, eczema, psoriasis)
- **Gastrointestinal system**: thrush, bloating, gas, intestinal cramps, rectal itching, alternating diarrhea and constipation
- **Genitourinary system**: vaginal yeast infections, frequent bladder infections
- **Hormonal system**: menstrual irregularities, PMS, menopause symptoms, fibroids, endometriosis
- **Nervous system**: depression, irritability, trouble concentrating, brain fog
- **Immune system**: allergies, chemical sensitivities, lowered resistance to infections, arthritis

The overuse of antibiotics as well as stressful conditions, damage to the intestinal tract, prescribed hormone treatments including birth control pills and hormone replacement therapy or immune system depression can all contribute to the overgrowth of Candida. Body processes are significantly disrupted as yeast cells and various toxic by-products of yeast metabolism easily enter general circulation.

Like most opportunistic infections, Candida overgrowth causes toxins to leak into the bloodstream or other tissues, allowing antigens (foreign substances) to invade bodily tissues. As an example a peanut is an antigen to a person who is allergic to peanuts. These antigens then trigger extensive allergic reactions which can lead to food, inhalant, and environmental allergies. The major waste product of yeast cell activity is Acetaldehyde, a poisonous toxin that promotes free radical activity in the body.

Yeasts cohabitate in a symbiotic relationship with over 400 healthy intestinal bacteria. These bacteria help produce short-chain fatty acids, vitamin K, biotin, vitamin B12, thiamin, and riboflavin. The yeast in the intestinal tract is kept in balance by these bacteria. Problems arise when the yeast flourish beyond healthy levels. This occurs when these good bacteria die from antibiotics or are suppressed by prescription steroids.

Acetaldehyde is the major breakdown by-product of yeast cell activity. This is a toxin that is poisonous because it promotes free radical activity within the body. Acetaldehyde is also converted by the liver into ethanol which is in drinking alcohol. There are many people with Candida that experience a feeling of intoxication, brain fogginess and a hung- over feeling along with debilitating fatigue from the high amounts of ethanol in their system.

Once the yeast organism invades and attaches itself to the intestinal walls, nutrition is compromised and the body is depleted of vital nutrients. In addition, over 79 distinct antigens have been clearly identified because of the large number of mycotoxins (substances naturally produced by fungus) and antigens secreted by Candida. The immune system is greatly taxed as a result of this overgrowth of Candida.

The History of Candida

A published article in 1978, written by Dr. C. Orian Truss stated that, "Tissue injury induced by Candida albicans: Mental and neurologic manifestations." (Journal of Orthomolecular Psychiatry, 7:1, 17:37, 1978.) described how Candida albicans, a yeast growing on the warm interior membranes of the body (including the digestive tract), could play an important role in problems throughout the body. Symptoms in patients with Candida-related health problems included fatigue, headache, PMS, depression and other disorders of the immune, endocrine and nervous systems.

Dr. Crook was skeptical at first when he investigated this article but many of his female patients seemed to fit Dr. Truss' hypothesis. So he contacted him about his findings. After communicating with Dr Truss, Dr Crook subsequently decided to prescribe to some of his own chronically ill patients a sugar-free diet along with the anti-fungal drug Nystatin. Dr Crook noted a dramatic improvement in the health of these patients. From this point on, Dr Crook began gathering data that documented this relationship between the overgrowth of Candida and health problems.

In December 1982, Dr. Crook introduced the concept of the "yeast connection" on a Cincinnati television show. Within a week, 7,300 letters arrived with requests for further information. This response led him to write The Yeast Connection, which was published in December 1983. This book has become a classic for people suffering from yeast-related problems.

Dr Crook knew that this theory would be slow to gain acceptance by the medical establishment. In 1986, the American Academy of Allergy and Immunology (AAAI) published a statement on what they called the

Candidiasis-Hypersensitivity Syndrome: "The concept is speculative and unproven; the basic elements of the syndrome could apply to almost all sick patients at some time. There is no published proof that Candida albicans is responsible for the syndrome." (J. Allergy Clin. Immunol., 1986; 78:271-273)

Despite criticism and occasional ridicule, Dr. Crook continued to believe in the validity of the relationship between yeast and human health. He diligently pursued his knowledge of Candida albicans and subsequently published a series of well-received books on the subject. In the late 1990s and into the 21st Century, new information about women's health problems appeared in both medical journals and the media.

CAUSES OF CANDIDA

A healthy body is by nature an unfriendly environment for harmful microorganisms. The normal acid-base balance of a well-functioning system does not generate a biochemical terrain in which Candida albicans or other parasitic infections can proliferate and thrive.

Candida albicans lives in all of our mucus membranes, i.e. intestines, eyes, ears, bladder, stomach, lungs, vagina, etc. It is one of the billions of other organisms that serve a useful purpose in the body. One of the important functions of Candida albicans is to recognize and destroy harmful bacteria and toxins. However, Candida is not intended to overgrow and get out of control while the body is still living because that change is only intended to happen when the body dies. At the point of death, Candida's functions and characteristics change for the purpose of breaking the body down. Candida releases substances, most of which are alcohols, which break down the body's tissues. When Candida overgrowth happens while the body is still alive, it causes innumerable symptoms, diseases and malfunctions.

Systemic yeast overgrowth or Candidiasis is not a condition acquired from some external source that can be effectively cured by the use of drugs. It is the result of living habits, dietary, environmental and even emotional influences that have led to a reduced level of biological functionality in the entire body as well as the mind and emotions in many cases. Yeast and other potentially harmful microorganisms would have no place to multiply out of control and mutate into pathogenic forms unless the proper conditions for their mutation and proliferation existed. Once the intestine's microbial ecology is sufficiently disturbed and the concentration of healthy bacterial species is greatly diminished, the Candida yeast organisms begin a process of mutation into harmful fungal forms. In their mutated forms, these fungal rhizoids develop elongated root-like structures which are capable of penetrating the intestinal lining as well as entering the circulating blood and colonizing tissues throughout the body. Such fungal organisms produce powerful toxins which severely challenge the system's detoxification pathways and enhance the symptoms of Candida.

Damage to the intestine's lining makes it more permeable to substances that were previously incapable of gaining entrance into the blood stream via the intestinal lining. Because of this phenomenon, aptly named "leaky gut syndrome", toxins and large food molecules which would normally have no way of getting into the circulating blood are absorbed. This creates an enormous burden on the immune system that now has to neutralize, destroy and eliminate the toxins. This produces many of the "allergic" and inflammatory symptoms that so often impact individuals with Candida overgrowth.

LISTED BELOW ARE THE MOST COMMON CAUSES OF CANDIDA.

1. ANTIBIOTICS

Antibiotics are a common cause of Candida. Antibiotics destroy both the harmful bacteria for which it is prescribed as well as the good bacteria that live in the gut. When antibiotics destroy the friendly bacteria, the Candida begins to multiply. This can leave your body defenceless to harmful bacteria and fungi such as the fast-growing Candida yeast that quickly dominates the small intestine and thus causes problems. Anyone who has been treated with antibiotics for acne, major dental work or any condition where antibiotic use has been frequent for more than a course of 7-10 days is a prime candidate for Candida.

2. POOR NUTRITIONAL CHOICES

The modern diet is like a feast for Candida because it is a yeast that needs sugar to thrive and multiply. Sugar itself is an issue along with foods containing sugar as well as anything that converts to sugar. The average person living in the western world consumes about 125 pounds of refined table sugar every year. Sugar is the main food supply of Candida. Refined carbohydrates such as processed food made with white flour including other refined grains as well as alcohol can all contribute to Candida growth.

A healthy immune system should be able to keep Candida at bay. However, a diet rich in sugar actually depresses your immune system, leaving it vulnerable and allowing the Candida yeast to proliferate.

3. BIRTH CONTROL PILLS OR DEVICES

Oral birth control pills are mostly comprised of the hormone estrogen. Supplemental estrogen in the synthetic form has been found to promote the growth of yeast. Several years ago the Great Smokies Medical lab published studies showing that hormones could affect intestinal bacteria. A common complaint of women on birth control pills is a yeast infection. The copper IUD is another possible yeast promoter. It has been observed by David Watts, Ph.D., that copper promotes the growth of yeast. Often copper IUD users develop excessive levels of copper in their tissues. Excess copper can depress the adrenal, thyroid and immune systems of the body which makes it more difficult for the body to resist yeast.

4. EXCESSIVE STRESS AND ELEVATED CORTISOL

Stress can cause yeast growth for several reasons. Stress causes the release of a certain hormone called cortisol. Elevated cortisol can depress the immune system and cause a rise in blood sugar. The Candida yeast feeds on the extra sugar while your weakened immune system is powerless to stop it. Quickly, it overpowers the balanced mixture of microorganisms in the small intestine. These two reactions tend to happen together as cortisol levels increase due to stress.

5. TAP WATER CONSUMPTION

Common tap water is high in chlorine which has been found to destroy friendly intestinal bacteria. This weakens your immune system and allows the small number of Candida yeast cells in your gut to grow into a Candida infestation. Most cities add chlorine to their drinking water. This means that you are drinking chlorine every day, bathing in it, showering in it, and using it to wash clothes. As a powerful disinfectant, chlorine ensures that the water supply stays free of pathogens. However the health benefits are out-weighed by chlorine's effect on your gut flora and immune system. Luckily there are ways to reduce your chlorine exposure. Using natural laundry products and regularly changing filters in the house result in less bodily exposure to this poisonous chemical.

6. PARASITES AND INTESTINAL WORMS

Some researchers have estimated that over 85% of all people living in North America and Canada have parasites. Parasites can be large worm-like creatures or small microscopic organisms. Either type destroys friendly bacteria in the intestines making yeast overgrowth possible. These parasites are a common human infestation in many parts of the world.

7. CONSTIPATION

Constipation can be caused by Candida. However constipation can also lead to Candida. If one does not have Candida and then becomes constipated for any reason, Candida may begin to grow. A digestive tract which is constipated is slow moving and becomes very alkaline. In order for Candida to thrive it requires an alkaline environment. The more alkaline the digestive tract, the happier the Candida becomes. It does not matter what causes the constipation. Constipation for any reason can easily cause Candida.

8. DRUGS AND ALCOHOL

Excess alcohol can directly destroy friendly bacteria and allow yeast to grow. Beer can be a particular problem not because of the yeast but because of its maltose content. Maltose is a sugar that is derived from malt. Malt sugar is very potent and can feed yeast cells very quickly. People with Candida also tend to develop allergies to all yeast products whether the yeast is healthy or not. This does not mean that hard spirits or wine in excess are any safer. Alcohol should always be used in moderation. Drugs can also cause yeast overgrowth particularly if they disturb the digestive system. Any medication or drug that can cause a gastrointestinal side effect may cause yeast growth by disturbing friendly bacteria. Steroid based drugs are a common cause of Candida.

9. HYPOTHYROID

Low thyroid is very common in cases of Candida. The thyroid gland has an important effect on the immune system. Adequate thyroid function also helps the digestive system to operate correctly. Lack of proper digestive secretions can cause reduction of friendly bacteria. Constipation is also common with low thyroid. Body temperature will drop if thyroid function is low. A drop in body temperature stops many different chemical reactions from taking place. Some of these chemical reactions stop Candida overgrowth.

10. IMMUNE DEFICIENCY

Any condition that results in a weakened immune system can bring about Candida. Most notable are AIDS and CANCER. Candida can be considered a side effect of these more threatening illnesses.

11. HORMONAL IMBALANCE

It has been long recognized that an imbalance between estrogen and progesterone can cause an overgrowth of yeast. In order to support friendly intestinal flora, adequate amounts of both hormones are needed. Any upset in this balance can cause yeast overgrowth. The hormonal imbalance must be corrected after the yeast has been reduced to avoid relapse.

12. DIABETES

It is extremely challenging to eliminate Candida while the blood sugar is high. Candida is just one of many conditions that Diabetes can bring about and diabetic women are particularly susceptible to any yeast infection. An elevated blood sugar level feeds the Candida yeast and allows it to grow quickly and it then dominates the other microorganisms in the gut.

13. THE TOXIC METAL CONNECTION

Toxic metals show up consistently in the candida patient. Silver amalgam fillings contain at least 50% mercury which is poisonous to the body. Mercury particles and vapor are continuously released in the body as you chew, grind and brush the teeth.

Mercury significantly weakens the immune system and can be the cause of many health problems. One of these is Candida. The mercury leaks from the dental fillings and kills the friendly bacteria in the gut and this allows Candida to take over. These metals disable the exact part of the immune system that seeks to control Candida! They are often found in dental fillings and in tap water. As they pass through the intestinal tract, they can stimulate the growth of more candida.

14. LACK OF HYDROCHLORIC ACID PRODUCTION

Hydrochloric acid, produced in the stomach, is a powerful defense against yeast because it activates pepsin in the gut and works to kill the harmful fungi in food. In addition, a lack of hydrochloric acid results in incomplete digestion resulting in the fermentation of carbohydrates. Fermented carbohydrates in the intestines promote yeast overgrowth. A common symptom for both bacterial and yeast overgrowth is the inability to tolerate the consumption of carbohydrates.

Any medication that reduces stomach acid levels can cause an overgrowth of Candida. The friendly bacteria, particularly acidophilus, release acid by-products that control the growth of Candida. The intestinal pH should be between 6.0 and 7.4. If the pH goes higher than 7.4, Candida begins to overgrow and establish colonies.

OTHER INFLUENCES THAT PREDISPOSE US TO CANDIDA ALBICANS OVERGROWTH AND MANY OTHER CHRONIC ILLNESSES
- Improper pre-natal and infant nutrition (both emotional & physical) such as a lack of or insufficiency of breast milk
- Introduction of animal proteins at too early an age produce life-long food allergies which lead to weakened immunity in childhood and adult life
- Consumption of de-mineralized, de-vitalized, and processed foods especially white sugar and white flour (the minerals in our foods allow the body to neutralize so many of the harmful acids that can accumulate in the system

- Consumption of chemical food additives, preservatives, stabilizers and coloring agents and artificial flavorings and sweeteners
- Commercially raised animal protein such as beef, chicken and farmed fish that contains trace amounts of antibiotics and/or artificial hormones
- Overeating, skipping meals on a regular basis, under eating, having coffee instead of breakfast, etc.
- Overuse of low quality fats, hydrogenated fats and trans-fatty acids such as margarine
- Insufficient amounts of fiber in the diet
- Drinking insufficient quantities of water to meet the body's requirements (8 fl. oz. / 250 ml. per 25 lbs. / 12 k. of body weight per 24 hours)
- Insufficient or excessive exercise, over-strenuous exercise for prolonged periods of time (excessive exercise weakens the body's defences; insufficient exercise lowers metabolic, circulatory & self-cleansing functions)
- Insufficient sleep, getting to sleep too late, shift work, frequent air travel through several time-zones (getting to sleep after 10 PM on a regular basis will deplete normal adrenal reserves and stress the entire system)
- Chronic stress
- Chemical contamination of work place and/or home
- Persons who handle or inhale chemical fumes / solvents in their work or hobbies
- Damp environments, mold and/or mildew in home, at workplace or in vehicles (ventilation ducts in the home or work place, as well as old car air conditioning systems often harbor considerable mold and mildew colonies; they should be cleaned regularly; filters should be changed more frequently than typically recommended)
- Living in proximity to commercial agricultural regions where agricultural chemicals are routinely sprayed
- Living in close proximity to high powered electric lines and other electromagnetic fields are disturbing influences
- Exposure/overexposure (there are no truly safe levels) to ionizing radiation
- Candida infection can be sexually transmitted and is most easily contracted by individuals with lowered immune functions

Symptoms of Candida

Candidiasis can present a wide variety of symptoms and the exact combination and severity of Candida related symptoms are unique to each individual case. Candidiasis can manifest itself through many seemingly unrelated symptoms and therefore the diagnosis is very often missed.

General Symptoms

- Inability to lose weight
- Water retention
- Weight loss
- Headaches
- Migraines
- Heart palpitations
- Cravings for sweets and alcohol
- Chronic fatigue

Psychological

- Inability to focus
- Poor memory
- Insomnia
- Persistent extreme fatigue
- Poor coordination
- Hyperactivity
- Anger
- Depression
- Crying spells
- Panic attacks
- Brain fog
- Irritability
- Sleep problems — difficulty falling asleep or waking up in the middle of the night with a mind that won't calm down (typically between 1 and 3 am)

- Dizziness
- Anxiety attacks, panic attacks
- Obsessive-compulsive disorder (OCD)
- Attention deficit, hyperactivity (ADD/ADHD)
- Numbness and tingling sensations
- Feeling of floating or not quite being in your body
- Indecisiveness, difficulty organizing and cleaning messy areas

DIGESTIVE SYSTEM

- Acid reflux
- Bloating
- Flatulence
- Nausea
- Diarrhea
- Constipation
- Stomach cramps
- Indigestion
- Belching after meals
- Mucus in stool
- Hemorrhoids
- Itching anus
- Irritable bowel syndrome
- Gas
- Abdominal pain
- Truncal obesity — excess weight centered around the abdomen
- Hypoglycemia (low blood sugar)

SKIN

- Acne
- Cysts
- Hives
- Night sweats
- Psoriasis
- Eczema
- Dermatitis
- Fungal infections of the nails and skin

- Athlete's foot
- Body odor
- Candida rash on the groin area
- Candida rash on the insides of ears
- Hair loss
- Prematurely graying hair
- Dilated pupils

ORAL

- Thrush (white coating on tongue)
- Swollen lower lip
- Halitosis
- Metallic taste in mouth
- Canker sores
- Bleeding gums
- Cracked tongue

RESPIRATORY SYSTEM

- Persistent cough
- Mucus in throat
- Sore throat
- Sinus congestion
- Chronic post-nasal drip
- Flu-like symptoms
- Hay fever symptoms
- Sinusitis
- Asthma

EYES AND EARS

- Eye pain
- Itchy eyes
- Sensitivity to light
- Blurred vision
- Dark circles under eyes
- Ringing in the ears
- Ear infections

GENITO-URINARY SYSTEM
- Recurring yeast infections
- Recurring UTI's (Urinary Tract Infections)
- Interstitial Cystitis (inflammation of the bladder)
- PMS (Pre Menstrual Syndrome)
- Menstrual irregularities
- Fungal rash
- Endometriosis
- Low libido

IMMUNE SYSTEM
- Frequent colds and flu
- Environmental allergies
- Food allergies
- Sensitivity to fragrances, chemicals and smoke
- Chronic Fatigue Syndrome
- Fibromyalgia
- Autoimmune conditions

MUSKULOSKELETAL
- Chronic body pain
- Joint pains
- Muscle aches and stiffness

Many experts agree that Candida is possibly the least understood and most widespread cause of chronic illness in modern day society. There are many people suffering from the symptoms of Candida without awareness that a single underlying cause could be to blame.

CHILDREN'S CANDIDA SYMPTOMS

Candida is well documented in pediatric health. Children can get yeast infections in all the classic ways. The white yeasty coat on the tongue or lips is known as thrush. Skin rashes including diaper rash, anal rash and even fungal sinus infections can all be linked to Candida. Fortunately children recover from Candida yeast overgrowths much faster than adults.

COMMON CANDIDA SYMPTOMS IN CHILDREN

- Frequent and heavy diaper rash
- Other "eczema" type skin rashes
- Oral thrush (white film in mouth or on lips or tongue)
- Colicky longer than 3 months
- Symptoms worse on damp days or in damp environments
- Recurrent ear problems
- Craving sweets all the time
- Headaches
- Hyperactive
- Learning problems
- Often irritable
- Ongoing nasal congestion, coughing or wheezing
- Unhappy, hard to please
- Seems unwell yet doctors do not find anything wrong

CAUSES OF CHILDHOOD CANDIDA

Frequent use of antibiotics for ear infections or steroids for the treatment of asthma or eczema can cause yeast in the intestinal flora to become unbalanced.

Children that experience baby thrush, cradle cap or chronic diaper rash have a higher tendency of developing other Candida related symptoms as they get older.

How Candida is formed in the Body

C andida Albicans is a negative yeast infection that begins in the digestive system and little by little spreads to other parts of the body. It is a strong, invasive fungus that attaches itself to the intestinal wall and can become a permanent resident in the internal organs. Candida may cause numerous health problems and discomfort for over 30 million men and women every day. It is estimated that many people have or will eventually have a moderate to serious condition of Candida.

About 80% of the time, candida overgrowth occurs when antibiotics kill the friendly bacteria in the intestinal tract. Overgrowth cannot occur when the immune system is strong and the friendly flora which is estimated to comprise 70% of the immune system response is plentiful.

When much of the friendly flora or bacteria have been destroyed and the immune system has weakened, the oxygen-loving Candida yeast begins to flourish. It then becomes an anaerobic Candida fungi. No longer needing an oxygen-rich blood supply, the fungi are able to exist anywhere in the body.

A yeast cell produces 79 known toxic substances that poison the human body including acetaldehyde which is the same chemical that causes a hang-over. These toxins contaminate the tissues, weakens the immune system, the glands, the kidneys, bladder, lungs, liver and especially the brain and nervous system. Candida yeast can become so massive and invasive that it progresses to the fungal form where it grows very long, root-like structures that penetrate the mucous lining of the gastrointestinal wall. This penetration breaks down the protective barrier between the intestinal tract and bloodstream, allowing many foreign and toxic substances to enter and pollute the body systemically. As a result, proteins and other food wastes that are not completely digested or eliminated can assault the immune system and can cause tremendous allergic reactions, fatigue and many other health problems. It also allows the Candida itself and bacteria to enter the bloodstream from which it may find its way to other tissues and this results in far-ranging effects such as soreness of the joints, chest pain, sinus and skin problems.

Candida yeast loves sugar and excretes chemicals that cause sugar cravings and all types of carbohydrates. As the yeast digests the food sugars before your body can use them, cravings may be caused by low blood sugar levels.

While sleeping at night, the body is in a fasting state and Candida has plenty of time to be consuming the body's blood sugar. To compensate for this lack of sugar, the adrenals have to work extra hard and this eventually leads to adrenal fatigue. The acetaldehyde produced by Candida also causes fatigue. The thyroid gland is linked with the adrenal glands. As the adrenal glands wear down, the thyroid gland also starts to perform poorly and this leads to decreased temperature regulation and low metabolism.

Candida covers the intestinal wall which chemically and mechanically interferes with digestion and assimilation of food nutrients. Many people, especially the elderly, cancer sufferers and those with AIDS are wasting away for want of nutrition because they cannot absorb what they eat. Many people digest less than 50% of their food because Candida may create a digestive conflict which robs the body of nutrition.

The major waste product of yeast cell activity is acetaldehyde, or ethanol. Many people have low iron in their blood because iron is hard to absorb when Candida is present and this deprives tissue of proper oxygenation. Ethanol may cause excessive fatigue and reduced strength and stamina. Ethanol destroys enzymes needed for cell energy and causes the release of free radicals that encourage the aging process.

Toxin Release

When the fungal levels in our bodies increase, we may experience symptoms such as nail fungus, vaginal yeast overgrowth, itchy skin, gas, bloating and sugar as well as carbohydrate cravings. Sufferers often describe a feeling of being worn-out and fatigued. This occurs when yeast overgrows in the body and it consumes the foods we eat for its own fuel and growth. As Candida overgrows, it releases toxic substances that cause a rundown feeling including somewhat foggy thinking. The multiplying colonies of yeast release acids that may render your internal environment more acidic. This increase in acidity often allows other harmful microorganisms to survive in the intestines, releasing more toxins and in turn compromising the body's health even further.

Candida also produces beta alanine which is a compound that interferes with the kidneys' reabsorption of the amino acid taurine. Interference with taurine metabolism can lead to lowered levels of magnesium and potassium as well as crucial electrolytes that maintain circulation and blood pressure. When the taurine supple is lowered, it can also disrupt the liver's detoxification functions leading to further depletion of the immune system.

WHY WOMEN HAVE SO MUCH MORE SERIOUS CANDIDA OVERGROWTH THAN MEN

Chronic Candida affects women approximately four times more often than men. The primary reasons that women are more affected are that women tend to be prescribed antibiotics more often for urinary tract infections and acne. Also, vaginal yeast infections have increased dramatically over the past 40 years due to many underlying factors. This increased incidence is mainly due to the increased usage of antibiotics. Other factors are also at work such as allergies, Diabetes mellitus, elevated vaginal pH, systemic Candida, the birth control pill, pregnancy and the use of steroids.

Some Estrogens will literally feed candida overgrowth and that is why birth control pills and estrogen replacement therapy put women at a greater risk of developing Candida overgrowth. Also, hormonal changes during the menstrual cycle can alter the pH of the vagina and the vaginal tract can be a very hospitable environment for Candida.

Candida blocks estrogen receptors so that estrogen can't lock into them. This further disrupts the endocrine hormone by binding to estrogen and this prevents it from being used properly by the body. Estrogen and progesterone should be in perfect harmony with each other but low estrogen levels can cause high progesterone levels. This imbalance creates low estrogen levels and the Candida causes progesterone levels to be elevated, providing more and more fuel for itself. Women often have flare-ups coinciding with their period because that is the time when progesterone levels are higher.

In addition to vaginal yeast infections, women with systemic Candida tend to suffer more severe forms of premenstrual tension or PMS. PMS is characterized by increasing symptoms 7-10 days before the onset of menstruation. Typical symptoms include fatigue, breast tenderness, irritability, depression, anxiety, headache or migraine, back pain, abdominal bloating, water retention and acne. It is estimated that 30-40% of women suffer from PMS with its peak occurrences among women between the ages of 30-40. Many women who overcome the systemic Candida often discover that their PMS is cured as well.

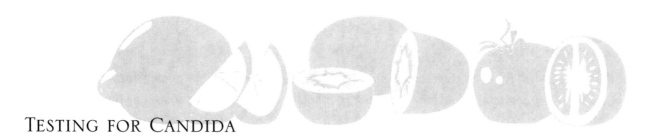

TESTING FOR CANDIDA

D iscovering if you have an overgrowth of Candida is crucial to overcoming any chronic condition. An excessive amount of Candida can destroy your health and quality of life in numerous ways. Many areas of the body can be affected such as the genital tract, digestive system, the heart, the brain, the liver, the joints and the eyes.

A Candida overgrowth has the ability to not only steal nutrients from the foods that you are consuming but also poison the tissues of the body with waste materials containing over 75 known toxins. The ravaging effects of this opportunistic yeast can manifest as numerous seemingly unrelated ailments.

As Candida flourishes, it plays into a larger problem called dysbiosis. Dysbiosis is the imbalance of the bacterial environment in the digestive tract. The army of "good" bacteria begins to dwindle because of poor dietary and lifestyle choices, stress, medications, and a weakened immune system. The result is that the "bad" bacteria then flourishes.

Many conventional medical practitioners do not recognize Candida as a medical issue. This makes it one of the most overlooked and chronic health issues this generation has had to face. Diagnosing Candida is not an easy task for any health practitioner due to the lack of agreement over a definitive diagnostic test for intestinal yeast overgrowth. However, there are many tests available to determine if the possibility of Candida exists. Step one is to begin with the Candida questionnaire.

CANDIDA QUESTIONNAIRE

A Candida self-test is one of the most useful and accurate methods of determining yeast-related health problems. It also serves as a tool for monitoring your health progress. Please answer all questions.

HISTORY		POINT SCORE
1. Have you taken tetracycline or other antibiotics for acne for one month or longer?		25
2. Have you, at any time in your life, taken other broad-spectrum antibiotics for respiratory, urinary or other infections for two months or longer or in short courses four or more times in a one-year period?		20
3. Have you ever taken a broad-spectrum antibiotic?		6
4. Have you been pregnant...?		
	One time?	3
	Two or more times?	5
5. Have you, at any time in your life, been bothered by persistent prostatitis, vaginitis, or other problems affecting your reproductive organs?		25
6. Have you taken birth control pills...?	For six months to two years?	8
	For more than two years?	15
7. Have you taken prednisone or other cortisone-type drugs...?		
	For two weeks or less?	6
	For more than two weeks?	15
8. Does exposure to perfumes, insecticides, fabric shop odors, and other chemicals provoke...		
	Mild symptoms?	5
	Moderate to severe symptoms?	20
9. Are your symptoms worse on damp, muggy days or in moldy places?		20
10.Have you had athlete's foot, ringworm, "jock itch," or other chronic infections of the skin or nails?		
	Mild to moderate?	10
	Severe or persistent?	20
11. Do you crave sugar?		10
12. Do you crave breads?		10
13. Do you crave alcoholic beverages?		10
14. Does tobacco smoke really bother you?		10

Total score of this section _____

MAJOR SYMPTOMS

For each of your symptoms, enter the appropriate figure in the point score column.

SCORE COLUMN

If a symptom is occasional or mild, score **3 points**.

If a symptom is frequent and/or moderately severe, score **6 points**.

If a symptom is severe and/or disabling score **9 points.**

POINT SCORE

1. Fatigue or lethargy _____

2. Feeling of being "drained" _____

3. Poor memory _____

4. Feeling "spacey" or "unreal" _____

5. Depression _____

6. Numbness, burning or tingling _____

7. Muscle aches _____

8. Muscle weakness or paralysis _____

9. Pain and/or swelling in the joints _____

10. Abdominal pain _____

11. Constipation _____

12. Diarrhea _____

13. Bloating _____

14. Persistent vaginal itch _____

15. Persistent vaginal burning _____

16. Prostatitis _____

17. Impotence _____

18. Loss of sexual drive _____

19. Endometriosis _____

20. Cramps and/or other menstrual irregularities _____

21. Premenstrual tension _____

22. Spots in front of the eyes _____

23. Erratic vision _____

TOTAL SCORE OF THIS SECTION _____

OTHER SYMPTOMS

For each of your symptoms, enter the appropriate figure in the point score column.

SCORE COLUMN

If a symptom is occasional or mild, score **1 point**

If a symptom is frequent and/or moderately severe, score **2 points**

If a symptom is severe and/or disabling, score **3 points.**

POINT SCORE

1. Drowsiness _____

2. Irritability _____

3. Lack of coordination _____

4. Inability to concentrate _____

5. Frequent mood swings _____

6. Headache _____

7. Dizziness/loss of balance _____

8. Pressure above ears, feeling of head swelling/tingling _____

9. Itching _____

10. Other rashes _____

11. Heartburn _____

12. Indigestion _____

13. Belching and intestinal gas _____

14. Mucus in stools _____

15. Hemorrhoids _____

16. Dry mouth _____

17. Rash or blisters in mouth _____

18. Bad breath _____

19. Joint swelling or arthritis _____

20. Nasal congestion or discharge _____

21. Postnasal drip _____

22. Nasal itching _____

23. Sore or dry throat _____

24. Cough _____

25. Pain or tightness in chest _____

26. Wheezing or shortness of breath _____

27. Urinary urgency or frequency _____
28. Burning on urination _____
29. Failing vision _____
30. Burning or tearing of eyes _____
31. Recurrent infections or fluid in ears _____
32. Ear pain or deafness _____

TOTAL SCORE OF THIS SECTION _____

TOTAL SCORE ALL SECTIONS _____

INTERPRETATION

	WOMEN	MEN
Yeast-connected health problems are almost certainly present	≥180	≥140
Yeast-connected health problems are probably present	120-180	90-140
Yeast-connected health problems are possibly present	60-119	40-89
Yeast-connected health problems are less likely present	≤60	≤40

LAB TESTING FOR CANDIDA

BLOOD TEST FOR CANDIDA

An immunoglobulin test measures the level of certain immunoglobulins or antibodies, in the blood. Antibodies are proteins made by the immune system to fight antigens such as bacteria, viruses, and toxins. IgA, IgG, and IgM are frequently measured simultaneously. Evaluated together, they can give health care practitioners important information about immune system functioning, especially relating to infection or autoimmune disease.

Blood analysis under powerful microscopes can be used to find Candida antibodies. When Candida takes on its fungal form, the immune system responds by producing special antibodies to fight off the infection. A large concentration of these antibodies in the blood is an indication of a Candidiasis overgrowth.

Candida Immune Complexes tests measure Candida specific IgG immune complexes. Immunoglobulin G (IgG), the most abundant type of antibody, is found in all body fluids and protects against bacterial and viral infections.

STOOL ANALYSIS FOR CANDIDA

The stool is directly analyzed for levels of yeast, pathogenic bacteria and friendly bacteria. Stool analysis tests diagnose Candidiasis through a laboratory examination of a stool sample. If the stool contains abnormally large amounts of Candida then Candidiasis may be indicated.

A stool analysis can also look at other digestive markers for determining Candida levels such as:
- Levels of beneficial bacteria in the intestines
- pH levels in the stool
- Intestinal parasites, like worms and single-celled organisms such as blastocystis hominis and amoeba
- SIgA which is the state of your gut immune system (a low SIgA can indicate low immunity or gut inflammation)
- Leaky gut syndrome

Urine Tartaric Acid Test

This test detects tartaric acid, a waste product of Candida yeast overgrowth. An elevated test means an overgrowth of Candida.

The Organic Acids Test (OAT)

The OAT provides an accurate evaluation of intestinal yeast and bacteria. Abnormally high levels of these microorganisms can be linked to behavior disorders, hyperactivity, movement disorders, fatigue and immune dysfunction. Many people with chronic illnesses and neurological disorders often excrete several abnormal organic acids. The cause of these high levels can include: oral antibiotic use, high sugar diets, immune deficiencies, and genetic factors.

Candida Urine Test

Secretory Immunoglobulin A (sIgA) test and intestinal permeability test can be taken to assess the permeability of the gut wall (leaky gut syndrome). This is associated with the development of food sensitivities and Candida infections in addition to a build up of potentially damaging toxins.

Breath Hydrogen Test

Bacterial dysbiosis results from the same causes as a Candida overgrowth. This is a test for bacterial overgrowth, or intolerances to lactose, fructose, or sucrose. The test measures the amount of hydrogen on a patient's breath within a specified amount of time after they have ingested a sugar solution. An elevated level of hydrogen indicates an overgrowth of bacteria in the small intestine. This test requires that you drink a solution of lactose, fructose, sucrose, or glucose in water.

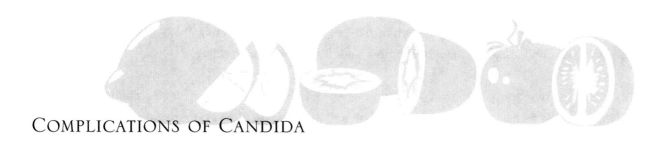

COMPLICATIONS OF CANDIDA

LEAKY GUT SYNDROME AND CANDIDA

Leaky Gut Syndrome is a weakening and inflammation of the intestinal wall. During Candida overgrowth, the yeast cells attach themselves to the intestinal walls, actually penetrating through the membrane into the bloodstream.

As Candida cells and food particles enter the circulatory system, they provoke a strong immune response from the body and this triggers an inflammatory response of the intestinal wall. These Candida cells and food particles are foreign particles that do not belong in the blood. The immune system reacts quickly to destroy them by sending specialized immune cells known as macrophages. Next, the immune system creates antibodies ready for the next time it sees these same cells. The next time this particular food is consumed, an immune response is triggered. This hypersensitivity of the immune system is how allergies start.

CANDIDA AND WEIGHT GAIN

One of the symptoms of systemic Candida is weight gain, or difficulty losing weight. It can cause the kind of stubborn fat deposits that are hard to shake off, no matter how little you eat or how much exercise you do. Candida cells are constantly reproducing and dying. The natural life cycle of this yeast results in toxins being released from dying Candida cells which are constantly being secreted into the bloodstream. The liver has to process these toxins and expel them from the body. If the liver becomes too burdened from too many toxins in the bloodstream, it has to accumulate these harmful chemicals to be processed later. This occurs because the liver stores them in fat cells primarily around the hips, belly and thighs. For many dieters, this is the root cause of abnormal fat deposits.

SUGAR CRAVINGS

Candida needs sugar to grow and reproduce. A typical symptom of a Candida infestation is increasingly severe sugar and carbohydrate cravings. The Candida yeast is consuming and burning large amounts of sugar and then sending blood sugar levels into hypoglycemia. This resulting low blood sugar triggers signals from your brain that you need to eat more and this results in overeating.

Once Candida overgrows in the large intestine where it is supposed to be in small amounts, it migrates upward into the small intestines where digestion and assimilation of all nutrients takes place. When the small intestine is overgrown with Candida, the digestion is inhibited because many of the beneficial bacteria in the small intestines that are needed for digestion as well as for your immune system are killed by the Candida.

Candida upsets the body's blood sugar as it seeks to be fueled by its primary food, sugar. Due to disrupted digestion by Candida, there is a lack of the minerals needed to escort sugar and insulin into the cells. This results in hypoglycemia as there are inadequate amounts of sugar entering the cells.

Due to the lack of minerals and low blood sugar tendencies which occur especially at night because the Candida has had a chance to burn through most of the sugar, the levels plunge even further. The brain then signals the adrenal gland to produce more adrenal hormones to keep the body functioning during the night. This can result in heightened cortisol and cause night sweats. The adrenal gland is now working overtime 24 hours per day and this leads to its eventual burn-out, resulting in adrenal fatigue. This depleted state of the adrenal glands further weakens the immune system leaving the body powerless and unable to fight Candida.

FACTS ABOUT CANDIDA

- Yeast secretes an enzyme that digests the lining of the intestines
- Yeast shifts the immune system from Th1 to Th2 (this sets the stage for allergies and viral infections)
- Yeast enzymes break down IgA (IgA is the most predominant type of antibody that is found covering the gut mucosa; IgA keeps toxins and bacteria from binding to the cells that line the intestines; without enough IgA, the intestines become inflamed, and the lymphoid tissue in the gut swells)
- The by-products of certain yeasts or fungus are able to alter the bacterial content of the intestines
- Candida secretes an enzyme that reduces the body's ability to kill Staphylococcus aureus which is a common pathogen in human intestines
- Yeast creates toxins like tartaric acid, acetaldehyde and arabinol that interfere with the body's ability to produce energy
- Yeast reduces the body's coenzyme Q10, coenzyme B6, alpha ketoglutaric acid, taurine and asparagine (these create a functional deficiency of B6, lipoic acid and folic acid)

According to Dr Gary Farr, the most harmful place for yeast seems to be in the small intestine. This was shown in a study of children with failure to thrive. Biopsies of the upper small intestine were taken and were examined with an electron microscope. The yeast was embedded in the intestinal lining in their invasive fungal or mycelial form. Some of these children had no yeast showing up in their stool. Yet the yeast in this first part of their intestinal tract was interfering with their nutrition.

The most documented proof of harmful yeast toxins come from the Great Plains Laboratory. Tartaric acid from yeast causes muscle weakness. Dr. Shaw discovered very high levels of tartaric acid in the urine of two autistic brothers. Both had such severe muscle weakness that neither could stand up. When treated with an antifungal called Nystatin, the tartaric acid measurements declined, and the children improved. When the Nystatin was discontinued, the tartaric acid levels rose, and the children got worse. Often, Dr. Shaw also finds tartaric acid in the urine of those with fibromyalgia which is a condition characterized by muscle pain, poor sleep and tender points.

CANDIDA DIE OFF REACTIONS

A Candida "Die-off" reaction (or a Herxheimer reaction) occurs when yeast cells are rapidly killed by the immune system or by an anti-fungal treatment program or an anti-Candida diet. This reaction is caused by the massive release of toxins from dying Candida cells. The Candida yeast cells actually release 79 different toxins when they die including ethanol and acetaldehyde. These toxic proteins from the dead yeast cells enter the bloodstream by crossing cell membranes and this activates an intense immune reaction.

Combinations of immune and yeast complexes initiate the release of histamine which is an irritating tissue hormone causing discomfort due to tissue inflammation. The symptoms of Candida are intensified through these severe allergic and toxic reactions.

Toxins released in the bloodstream can strain the eliminative capacities of the liver, kidneys, colon and lymphatic system as they make their way out of the body, producing uncomfortable symptoms. The body goes through several processes of detoxification to eliminate the burden released by dead and dying yeast cells. The elimination of dead yeast cells is a progressive and ongoing process carried out by the elimination organs of the body.

Many systems of detoxification are affected as the cells and tissues begin to eliminate the waste and carry it from the bloodstream to various areas including the bowels, kidneys, lungs, skin, nasal passages, ears, throat, and genital organs. These structures in turn become over-polluted producing symptoms such as nausea, diarrhea, colds, kidney and bladder infections, headaches, skin irritation, fatigue and fevers.

Many people can tolerate the Candida die-off symptoms and general reactions to the cleansing process can be minimal. The important thing to remember is if you are experiencing a moderate to severe reaction is to continue on with the cleansing protocol because the die-off symptoms will lessen quickly. These die-off reactions usually settle within a week but may last up to a few weeks. There are several coping strategies to be taken into consideration (see below for strategies).

DIE-OFF SYMPTOMS

Here is a list of some of the symptoms you might experience during a die-off:
- Nausea
- Headache, fatigue, dizziness
- Swollen glands
- Bloating, gas, constipation or diarrhea
- Increased joint or muscle pain
- Elevated heart rate or heart palpitations
- Chills, cold feeling in your extremities
- Body itchiness, hives or rashes
- Sweating
- Fever
- Skin breakouts
- Recurring vaginal, prostate and sinus infections
- Brain fog
- Poor concentration
- Tightness in the chest
- Sore throat
- Anxiety
- Depression
- Irritability
- Feeling sick all over
- Intense cravings for sweets and carbohydrates
- Cravings for alcohol

COPING WITH CANDIDA DIE-OFF
- Take herbs such as Milk thistle, Dandelion root, Burdock root or Blue flag that help your to liver eliminate the toxins
- Molybdenum is a trace mineral that is helpful for counteracting die-off symptoms because it converts the neurotoxin acetaldehyde into acetic acid, which is then expelled by your body or even converted into helpful digestive enzymes
- Reducing or eliminating the amount of anti-fungal supplements in your program will diminish the die-off symptoms (as your symptoms lessen you can increase the dose slowly back up to the full prescribed amount)

- Probiotics are less likely than antifungals to cause die-off reactions, but if you start to experience the symptoms you can temporarily reduce your dosage until you are able to slowly increase (a course of good probiotics will repopulate your gut, crowd out the Candida, restore your stomach acidity and boost your immune system)
- Increase your consumption of water (4-6 fluid ounces of warm or hot water every forty-five minutes, throughout the day will encourage the elimination of toxins)
- Rest is an essential part of decreasing the die-off symptoms (neglecting to rest can potentially cause the reactions to be aggravated)
- Take 1000 mg of Vitamin C at least twice daily or to bowel tolerance (take 1000 mg of Vitamin C every hour until the bowels become loose then lessen the dose by 1000 mg).
- Adhere to the specific dietary anti-Candida restrictions (straying from the diet will only strengthen the opportunistic Candida; if you've cut out all grains from your diet and are experiencing yeast die-off reactions, the re-introduction of a small amount of brown rice or quinoa can be beneficial)
- Take your time at meals and chew food slowly and completely
- Include a variety of healthful, fresh vegetables on a daily basis
- Ensure you are having regular bowel movements
- Increase fibre and water intake to optimize bowel function
- Take short walks to stimulate circulation
- Use an infrared sauna to promote lymphatic drainage and detoxification (begin slowly- 20 minutes per session and increase up to 45 minutes; shower immediately afterwards)
- Have Epsom salt baths—20 minute soak in 1-2 cups of Epsom salts per tub full of hot water; shower off after bath
- Do daily dry skin brushing with a dry loofah; brush in circular motions always towards the heart
- Try a contrast shower (5 minutes warm water followed by 1 minute cold water)
- Healthy bowel function enhances the elimination of toxins (three bowel movements per day are ideal; if you are constipated or eliminating less than three times per day)
- The following are some steps to enhance bowel function:
    - Use Magnesium citrate before bed at a dose of 150mg- 750mg (start with the lower dose and increase as needed)
    - Start every morning with a tall glass of very hot water and half the juice of one lemon
    - Add 2 tablespoons of ground flax to your diet (add to plain yogurt or a smoothie)
    - Consume ½ cup of aloe vera juice each day to facilitate the bowels
    - Take an extra dose of probiotics before bed
    - Administer a warm, salt-water enema or a coffee enema to greatly encourage the bowels
    - Never ignore the urge!

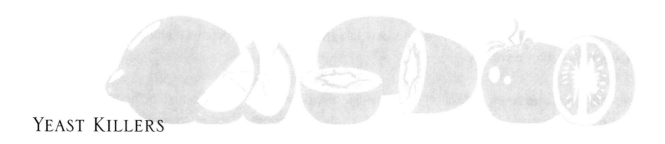

Yeast Killers

Antifungals are equally as important as probiotics in the fight against Candida. In fact, antifungals and probiotics work synergistically to kill off the yeast and restore a healthy balance to the digestive system. Antifungals kill the Candida yeast and then the probiotics replenish your gut with good bacteria to prevent the Candida from overgrowing again.

Plant-derived antifungal medications are a very effective way to kill off Candida. Some plants have naturally occurring antifungal plant chemicals in them. As plants extend their roots into wet soil, fungal invasion and eventual rot are constant threats to the life of a plant. Nature, therefore, endows plants with antifungal chemicals that course through their tubules (their circulatory system) and successfully keep fungi at bay. When this system breaks down like when a plant is damaged or diseased, plants break apart and soften up as fungus invades. This becomes easier to understand when picturing a rotting tree with mushrooms growing on the remaining bark.

Just as fungal chemicals from nature (antibiotics like penicillin) are effective agents for killing bacteria, man can also use plant chemicals from nature to kill fungus. Currently, none of the synthetic medications appear to work as well as plant-derived antifungals for Candida overgrowth.

There are many effective natural antifungals that can be used in the treatment of Candida. The following is a list of the most clinically proven methods of eradicating Candida:

Natural Antifungal Treatments

Bentonite Clay

Bentonite Clay is a detoxifying agent with some unique properties. It contains charged particles which bind to toxins in your gut. Bentonite clay cannot be absorbed into the body, so these toxins then pass through the gut and leave your body. Natural Sodium Bentonite clay is known traditionally for its use in the treatment of mineral deficiencies. It helps in binding the harmful toxic elements and makes them more soluble. It absorbs heavy metallic elements, impurities and certain other bodily contaminants. Mineral deficiencies such as anemia, abdominal ulcers, diarrhea, intestinal problems, hemorrhoids etc are also treated using this kind of clay.

Bentonite provides strong detoxification in the digestive tract. It has the ability to bind herbicides, viruses and other potentially harmful substances by its absorbent action. Bentonite's mechanism of action is physical due to its colloidal structure and charged particles which allow it to bind with toxins in the stomach, small intestine and colon. It is not digested nor is it absorbed into the bloodstream. Since toxins are bound to the bentonite, they are excreted from the body when the bentonite is eliminated through bowel movements.

SUGGESTED ADULT USE: For daily use, take 1 tablespoonful with liquid once per day on an empty stomach early in the morning or late at night. Drink additional fluid during the day. Mix with 1 teaspoon of psyllium or apple pectin for additional binding.

NOTE: Make sure the bentonite clay does not come into contact with any metals as it will deactivate the clay.

Caprylic Acid

Caprylic Acid is one of the three fatty acids (along with capric acid and lauric acid) that are found in coconut oil. It is a potent antifungal that kills Candida cells and it also restores stomach acidity to normal levels.

Like other antifungals, caprylic acid works by interfering with the cell walls of the Candida yeast. Repeated studies have shown its effectiveness against Candida. According to a study conducted by Japan's Niigata University, "the fungicidal effect of caprylic acid on Candida Albicans was exceedingly powerful". Caprylic acid also helps to normalize the acidity in your stomach. Candida dieters are frequently confused as to whether they should be trying to make their stomach more alkaline or more acidic. This confusion is caused because the stomach naturally has a much higher acidity than the rest of your body. Stomach acidity is important because it allows your immune system to function properly, enabling it to fight off the Candida overgrowth. Caprylic Acid helps to restore a natural, acidic environment to your stomach.

SUGGESTED ADULT DOSE: 1000 mg 3 times per day 20 minutes before a meal.

Coconut Oil

Coconut oil is often recommended as an adjunct to the Candida diet because of its special antimicrobial properties. Coconut oil is rich in saturated fats, especially medium-chain fatty acids, or MCFAs, from which everybody, especially Candida sufferers, can benefit. The MCFAs specifically found in coconut oil are called caprylic acid, capric acid and lauric acid. The special structure of these fatty acids allows them to attack the integrity of the membrane of Candida yeast, disrupting and disintegrating it, which leaves the interior of its cell, called the cytoplasm, disorganized and shrunken, as explained by researchers of the University of Iceland responsible for the study. This has been shown to kill Candida yeast without leading to the development of more resistant Candida strains observed with other antifungal treatment

Coconut oil is a tremendously versatile antifungal that is really easy to add to your diet. You can take by the spoon as a supplement or just use it as a replacement for other cooking oils.

As an entirely natural antifungal, coconut oil is a safe and effective way to prevent your Candida over-growth from returning. Make it a part of your long term diet plan and you will find it has many other health benefits besides its antifungal properties. Even better, combine it with other coconut-based products like coconut flour for baking and coconut aminos for salad dressings and as a substitute for soy sauce.

Adding coconut oil to your diet can be as quick and easy as taking 1-2 tablespoons of the oil each morning. If you don't recognize any die-off symptoms, increase your dose gradually up to 5 tablespoons daily. Alternatively, you can use coconut oil as a substitute for other oils in your cooking. Coconut oil is very heat-stable oil which means that it does not break down into unhealthy trans fats when it is cooked to high temperatures.

SUGGESTED ADULT DOSE: 1-5 tablespoons per day.

BERBERINE

Berberine is an alkaloid found in an herb called Barberry (Berberis vulgaris). It is also found in related plants Goldenseal, Oregon grape root and Chinese goldthread. This herb has long been used in Chinese and Ayurveda medicine. Berberine has significant antifungal activity and is also effective against some kinds of bacteria. Berberine is reported to spare beneficial organisms such as lactobacilli species. An added benefit for some people is its antidiarrheal action. Research has shown that Berberine can effectively prevent Candida species from producing an enzyme called lipase which they use to help them colonize. Berberine has also been widely shown to have a powerfully direct antifungal action.

SUGGESTED ADULT DOSE: 1 capsule two to three times per day

OIL OF OREGANO

The wild Oregano shrub originates high in the Mountains of the Mediterranean where its medicinal properties have been known for centuries. Indeed, it has long been used as a natural alternative to antibiotics.

Oregano vulgare contains a variety of substances that make it an effective antifungal. In a study assessing its action against Candida Albicans, carvacrol, a major phenolic constituent of the oil, was found to inhibit Candida to a greater extent than caprylic acid. It is also highly effective against many bacteria with studies published in the most prestigious medical journals which showed that it is as effective as many antibiotic drugs. Another study demonstrated its potency against parasites and worms which makes it a useful supplement for those Candida sufferers who also have Leaky Gut Syndrome. It also has antioxidant properties. One advantage that Oregano oil has over other antifungals is that the Candida yeast does not develop resistance. Some other antifungals may lose their effectiveness over time as the Candida adapts to them.

Oil of Oregano can either be used to treat topical fungal infections or taken orally in a capsule or liquid form.

SUGGESTED ADULT DOSE: 1-6 drops under the tongue per day. Start with 1 drop and slowly work up to a maximum dose of 6 drops. Alternatively, oil capsules containing 181mg of Oregano oil can be taken at a dosage of 1 cap 2 times per day after a meal to a maximum dose of 2 caps 2 times per day after a meal.

GARLIC

Garlic (Allium sativum) contains a large number of sulphur containing compounds that exhibit potent antifungal properties. Among the most studied are allicin, alliin, alliinase and S-allylcysteine. Some studies have found garlic to be at least as effective as Nystatin at killing Candida albicans. One of the key compounds in garlic is ajoene which is a proven antifungal that has been shown to be effective against many fungal strains. Ajoene is formed from a compound named allicin and an enzyme named allinase. When these two natural compounds come into contact by chopping the garlic, crushing it or by other means, they form an antibacterial agent named allicin which then combines to form ajoene. Although this has proven antifungal properties, the exact mechanism by which this happens is not clear. As with other antifungals, scientists suspect that it works by disrupting the walls of the cells of the Candida yeast cells.

Garlic has a long history of medicinal use which dates as far back as 3000 years. For treating intestinal yeast infections, garlic is available in a number of different forms including odorless capsules, liquid extract and tablets. However, a study at the National Institutes of Health found that fresh garlic was significantly the most potent against Candida albicans. Therefore adding raw garlic to or crushing and swallowing raw cloves if you can tolerate it is a cheap and powerful anti-fungal treatment.

SUGGESTED ADULT DOSE:

Garlic cloves: 2 to 4 grams per day of fresh, minced garlic cloves

Garlic Tablets: 600 to 900 mg daily, freeze-dried garlic standardized to 1.3% alliin or 0.6% allicin

Garlic Oil: 0.03 to 0.12 mL three times a day

COLLOIDAL SILVER

Silver is a well-known antimicrobial. It is commonly used in items such as water filters to kill any microbe that may be in the water such as bacteria, fungi, worms and protozoa. Colloidal silver is a suspension of silver particles in water. Colloidal silver is proven to be effective against up to 650 pathogens including yeast and fungi species as well as Candida. The colloidal silver provides a three-fold attack on the problems of Candida. First, the colloidal silver kills off anaerobic bacteria and viruses wherever it comes in contact with them. Therefore, the colloidal silver virtually provides a secondary immune system against all types of disease and infections while treating the Candida. Thus much of the problems of Candida are treated immediately before the Candida can be cleaned out of the system. Second, colloidal silver is unusually effective in treating the Candida infection itself. It works by denaturing the enzyme involved with supplying the organism with oxygen. Thirdly, colloidal silver has a strange and dynamic way of healing injured and damaged tissues quickly. Since yeast infections of all kinds usually attack and consume the living tissue, a healing process is badly needed and colloidal silver has a very unique way of healing these tissues quickly.

SUGGESTED ADULT DOSAGE

Internally: 1 tsp. three times per day- hold under the tongue for 30 seconds and swallow

Externally: Apply topically up to 4 times per day to affected areas (i.e. athletes foot, toenail fungus, vaginal yeast infections and fungal related rashes)

BLACK WALNUT

Black walnut contains a high amount of plant tannins making it an effective natural antifungal. Tannins are responsible for the sharp and biting taste of red wines like merlots and cabernets. They are also found in the bark of trees that are particularly resistant to fungus such as the Redwood tree. Tannins are available in a number of forms to treat intestinal yeast overgrowth. In a 1990 University of Mississippi study, the active ingredient in Black walnut (juglone) was shown to be as effective as some commercial antifungals. According to the study, the test results for juglone have repeatedly shown it to have moderate antifungal activity and to be as effective as certain commercially available antifungal agents such as zinc undecylenate and selenium sulfide.

SUGGESTED ADULT DOSAGE: Black walnut liquid extract made from the husk or hulls- 0.5 mls 3 times per day

GRAPEFRUIT SEED EXTRACT

Grapefruit Seed Extract (GSE) comes from the pulp and seeds of grapefruit. A 2004 study showed that GSE inhibited the growth of Candida Albicans and this is one of the most popular antifungals used for cases of Candida overgrowth.

In another 1990 study, grapefruit seed extract was found to perform as well or better than 30 antibiotics and 18 fungicides all without side effects. This study of grapefruit seed extract that was published in the Journal of Orthomolecular Medicine found GSE to be highly effective against different yeasts and molds such as Candida, Geotrichum, Aspergillus and Penicillium species. GSE's antifungal properties help it to combat Candida infestations by killing the yeast cells that have multiplied throughout the intestines.

Grapefruit seed also contains important nutrients such as Vitamins C & E and plant bioflavonoids. These can all help to repair the cells in the body that are destroyed by the Candida. One particular bioflavonoid named Hesperidin has immune boosting properties. The natural acidity of the extract also helps your immune system by restoring your stomach to its natural pH as it can frequently become too alkaline during Candida overgrowth.

SUGGESTED ADULT DOSAGE: 10 drops of the liquid extract in a cup of water 3 times a day. In tablet form, 100-200mg 3 times a day.

PROBIOTICS

Probiotics are an absolutely essential part of any Candida fighting program. Probiotics serve many purposes in the body and help to build up the immune system. The immune system is a complex network of many different organs and systems in the body. Researchers are still discovering how these different areas of the immune system work together to protect the body from disease. The digestive tract is one of the main players in a healthy functioning immune system. It actually comes down to the balance between the beneficial and pathogenic bacteria within the digestive system that dictate the health of the immune system.

There have been several studies that have shown that probiotics help support the immune system in its protection against pathogens of all types. A 2009 study at the University of Pennsylvania found that a healthy balance of bacteria in the gut will actually boost the immune system. The study also showed that normal levels of bacteria actually increase the effectiveness of the immune system and help the body to fight off pathogens. Another paper by the Yale Group in 2008 found that probiotics might be of value for incorporation into the daily diet of healthy people for the purpose of staying healthy.

Without a healthy immune system, the fight against Candida will be ruthless. Probiotics have also been shown to prevent the recurrence of Candida by continuing with them after the Candida cleanse is completed.

Probiotics have many other direct benefits in the elimination of Candida. The beneficial bacteria contained in probiotics secrete small quantities of lactic acid and acetic acid. These help to maintain the correct levels of acidity in your stomach. Candida yeast can switch to its pathogenic, fungal form in an alkaline environment and thus returning the stomach to its normal acidity will restrain the Candida overgrowth.

The stomach can become too alkaline in a number of ways but the most common cause is antibiotic intake. A course of antibiotics kills all the bacteria in your stomach and many of these probiotics like acidophilus are acid-producing. Ordinarily the acidity level in the stomach should be between 1 and 2 on the pH scale while conversely the blood pH should be between 7.35 and 7.45 which make it much more alkaline. This high level of acidity in the stomach helps with digestion and is one of the best defenses against pathogens like Candida Albicans.

During treatment for Candida overgrowth, it is essential that probiotic bacteria are consumed concurrently to restore the proper balance of organisms in the gut. When undergoing antifungal treatment, the pathogenic organisms are killed off and therefore space within the intestines and along the intestinal wall becomes available for colonization by other organisms. Taking probiotic supplements enhances the chances of these new colonies being made up of beneficial bacteria rather than of pathogenic types. Also of importance to sufferers of environmental illnesses is the fact that recent research has shown that the gut flora is directly linked to the development of allergies to both food and airborne allergens. Therefore improving gut flora could potentially reduce the number and severity of allergies that are often seen in the Candida sufferer.

TYPES OF PROBIOTIC BACTERIA

The most numerous probiotic bacteria normally inhabiting the small intestine are species of Lactobacilli. In the colon the majority are mainly Bifidobacteria. Most probiotic products consist of one or more species of bacteria from one or both of these types.

GENERAL BENEFITS OF LACTOBACILLI:
- Prevent overgrowth of disease-causing microbes: Candida species, E. coli, Helicobacter pylori (H. pylori), and Salmonella
- Prevent and treat antibiotic-associated diarrhea
- Aid in digestion of lactose and dairy products
- Improve nutrient absorption
- Maintain integrity of the intestinal tract and protect against macromolecules entering the bloodstream and causing antigenic responses
- Lessen intestinal stress from food poisoning
- Acidify intestinal tract (low pH provides a hostile environment for pathogens and yeast)
- Helps prevent vaginal and urinary tract infections

GENERAL BENEFITS OF BIFIDOBACTERIA:
- Prevent colonization of the intestine by pathogenic bacteria and yeasts by protecting the integrity of the intestinal lining
- Produce acids that keep the pH balance in the intestine (this acid environment prevents disease-producing microbes from getting a foothold)
- Decrease the side-effects of antibiotic therapy
- Primary bacteria in infants which helps infants grow
- Inhibit growth of bacteria that produce nitrates in the bowel (nitrates are bowel toxic and can cause cancer)
- Help prevent production and absorption of toxins produced by disease-causing bacteria which reduces the toxic load on the liver
- Aids in the manufacture of B-complex vitamins

- Help regulate peristalsis and bowel movements
- Prevent and treat antibiotic-associated diarrhea

(Source: <u>Digestive Wellness</u> by Liz Lipski, Ph.D., CCN)

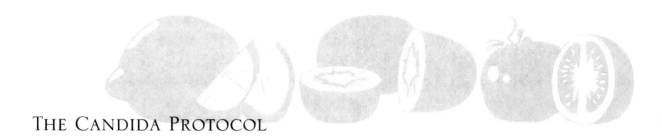

THE CANDIDA PROTOCOL

Once a Candida diagnosis has been confirmed through the Candida questionnaire and/or one of the recommended lab tests, the protocol can begin for a minimum of three months. For the elimination of Candida to be successful, strict adherence to the plan is crucial. Candida is an opportunistic fungus and it will strike and flourish at any opportunity. The weakest strains are killed off initially and the stronger strains take more time to be eliminated. Therefore any variance while on the plan will only serve to strengthen the stronger strains of Candida which then render it much more difficult to treat.

DIETARY GUIDELINES

Follow the dietary guidelines outlined in the "Do's and Don'ts" Food Lists.

Month 1- In addition to the dietary guidelines, eliminate all grains in all of their forms for a period of one month. After one month, only 1 cup of gluten free whole grains per day can be reintroduced. In some cases complete elimination of grains is needed throughout the cleansing period. If after 1 month of the plan there is not a complete elimination of symptoms, it is then recommended to remain grain free for the duration. No flour of any grain is allowed during the entire program. If grains are tolerable after the month elimination, then only whole grains are permitted (ie whole brown rice is allowable but brown rice flour is not).

SUPPLEMENTS

all recommended supplements are available online at www.drcobi.com

During the Candida Protocol, the antifungals will be rotated each month to prevent any resistance to occur. Candida has a tendency to become familiar with certain antifungals causing them to stop working. Alternating the remedies each month will ensure that does not occur.

Choose one of the antifungals each month and take the full recommended dose. If any "die off" reactions occur during the first few weeks, decrease the dose by half and slowly work back up to the full dose. You can also utilize the remedies under the "die off" support list to help ease the detoxification symptoms.

ANTIFUNGALS:

Caprylex (Douglas labs) (*Contains Caprylic acid*)–Take 1 to 3 tablets three times daily with food

Berbercap (Thorne) (*Contains Berberine HCl*)–Take 1 capsule two to three times daily with food

Anti-MFP (Douglas Labs)(*Contains: Grapefruit Seed Extract, Olive Leaf Extract, Berberine HCl, Burdock (root), Goldenseal (root), Black Walnut Hull Powder*) -Take 2 to 4 capsules daily with food

Grapefruit seed extract –Take 10 to 20 drops of liquid or 200 mg of powder or pills three times daily with food

Yeast Balance Complex (Integrative Therapeutics)(*Contains a comprehensive blend of Goldenseal, Pau d'arco, Milk thistle, Garlic, Barberry, Prebiotics, Probiotics and digestive enzymes*) -Take 1-2 caps three times daily with food

Formula SF722 (Thorne) (*Contains Undecylenic acid–from Castor beans*) -Take 5 gel caps three times daily with food

Candibactin AR (Metagenics) (*Contains Red Thyme oil, Oregano oil, Sage leaf, Lemon balm*)–Take 1 softgel three times daily with food

Candibactin BR (Metagencis) (*Contains Coptis, Oregon grape, Berberine HCl, Chinese skullcap, Phellodendron bark, Gingerrhizome, Chinese licorice root, Chinese Rhubarb root and rhizome*)- Take 2 tablets two to three times daily with food

Oil of Oregano- 4–6 drops (about 50 mg. of 100% pure Oil of Oregano diluted with a carrier oil such as olive oil. A safe blend is 1 part oregano oil to 3 parts olive oil)–can also be used topically for yeast related rashes and infections

Pleo-Ex (Sanun)- 5-10 drops one time per day

OTHER SUPPORTIVE ANTIFUNGALS WHICH CAN BE USED IN ADDITION TO THE ABOVE MENTIONED REMEDIES:

Coconut oil- Start with 1 teaspoon per day and work up to 5 teaspoons per day -can also be used topically for yeast related rashes and infections

Colloidal silver- Hold 1 teaspoon under the tongue for thirty seconds and swallow -can also be used topically for yeast related rashes and infections (do not use internally for longer than 30 days consecutively)

Bentonite Clay- It is generally advisable to start with 1 tablespoon of bentonite clay daily mixed with a small amount of water (pay attention to the results for a week and then gradually increase the dosage to no more than 4 tablespoons daily in divided doses)

Psyllium powder- 1/2 to 2 tsp of psyllium powder into 8 oz. of water (drink an additional 8oz of water to prevent constipation from occurring)

Allium sativa (garlic) -An encapsulated supplement is sometimes necessary to deliver high enough concentrations to the intestines which will avoid irritating the stomach (also beneficial is to include one to three cloves of raw garlic in the diet daily)

PROBIOTICS

Probiotics play a critical role in the elimination of Candida. The term 'probiotic' is derived from the Greek, meaning 'for life'. Probiotics are currently defined as 'live microorganisms which, when consumed in adequate amounts, confer a health benefit to the host. Common descriptions for probiotics include 'friendly', 'beneficial' or 'healthy' bacteria.

The beneficial bacteria contained in probiotics secrete small quantities of lactic acid and acetic acid. These help to maintain the correct levels of acidity in your stomach. This is important because the Candida yeast can switch to its pathogenic, fungal form in an alkaline environment, therefore restoring the stomach back to its normal acidity will restrain the Candida overgrowth.

It is crucial to take Probiotics daily without food throughout the entire protocol. Probiotics are best taken before bed or first thing in the morning with a full glass of non-chlorinated water. Lactobacilli are probably the most important addition to the diet in combating a gastrointestinal yeast overgrowth. Both are taken by mouth or as rectal implants. Two strains are of significance Lactobacillus acidophilus (especially for upper GI) and Bifidobacterium bifidus (especially for the colon or large bowel).

Ultraflora Balance (Metagenics) (*Contains a dairy free patented probiotics blend of 15 billion of B.lactis Bi-07 and L. acidophilus NCFM which is the most well researched probiotic strain*) -Take 1 capsule one to two times per day on an empty stomach

Ultra Flora IB (Metagenics) (*Contains 60 billion strain-identified micro-organisms in a 50:50 ratio including B.lactis Bi-07 and L. acidophilus NCF)*–Take 1 capsule one to two times daily on an empty stomach

Sacro B (Saccharomyces boulardii) (Thorne) (*Contains a yeast species that can provide substantial support to the health of the gastrointestinal tract by supporting beneficial intestinal flora)* -Take 2 capsules two times daily on an empty stomach

Multi Probiotic 4000 (Douglas Labs)–*(Contains a combination of 15 billion organisms coming from 6 different strains and a pre-biotic blend)*–Take 1 to 2 capsules two time daily on an empty stomach

HMF Series Probiotics (Genestra):

HMF Candigen (*Contains two strains of Lactobacillus and garlic in a vaginal ovule form)*–Use 1 ovule per day at bedtime

HMF Candigen Cream-150 billion CFU per dose (*Contains two strains of Lactobacillus, Garlic and Rosa Damascena in a cream form)*–Apply a thin layer of cream to the external vaginal area two to three times daily

HMF Replete (*Contains a highly concentrated probiotic formula of two strains of Lactobaccillus acidophilus, Lactobacillus salivarius, Bifidobacterium bifidum and Bifidobacterium animalis lactis along with fructooligosaccharides)* -Take one sachet per day for 7 days on an empty stomach

HMF Replenish-100 billion CFU per dose (*Contains two strains of Lactobaccillus acidophilus, Lactobacillus salivarius, Bifidobacterium bifidum and Bifidobacterium animalis lactis along with fructooligosaccharides)* -Take 1 capsule daily on an empty stomach

HMF Intensive- 25 billion (*Contains two strains of Lactobaccillus acidophilus, Lactobacillus salivarius, Bifidobacterium bifidum and Bifidobacterium animalis lactis)* -Take 1 capsule per day on an empty stomach

SUPPORTIVE NUTRIENTS

all recommended supplements are available online at www.drcobi.com

The following is a list of supportive nutrients that can be taken throughout to give additional healing benefits to the immune system, digestive system and liver function.

DIGESTIVE SUPPORT

The body uses stomach acid and enzymes secreted from the stomach and pancreas to break down large molecules for proper absorption through the intestinal wall into the bloodstream. Incomplete digestion of proteins and other food components leads to food sensitivities and the formation of toxic substances. These powerful enzymes also keep the intestines free from parasites, including yeast. To aid the body in this process, the following may be recommended:

HYDROCHLORIC ACID:

BPP enzymes (Thorne) (*Contains a blend of HCl, pepsin and pancreatin)* –Take 1 to 2 capsules with meals daily

Bio-Gest (Thorne) *(Contains a blend of HCl, pepsin, pancreatin and ox bile)* –Take 1 to 2 capsules with meals daily

Dipan-9 (Thorne) *(Contains pancreatin and a blend of lipase, protease and amylase)* –Take 1 to 2 capsules with meals daily

PANCREATIC ENZYMES:

Ultrazyme (Douglas labs) (*Contains a full spectrum, high potency enzyme supplement specifically formulated with bovine bile extract and high levels of active pancreatic enzymes)*–Take 1 or 2 tablets with meals daily

GI Digest (Douglas Labs)- *(Contains a plant based full spectrum enzyme supplement with amylase, protease, lipase, cellulose and lactase)*–Take 1 to 2 caps with meals daily

L-Glutamine powder (Thorne)–Take 5 grams per day dissolved in water or a smoothie

IMMUNE SUPPORT

Vitamin D3- Critical for immune system support – Adults take 2000 IU-5000 IU per day

Vitamin A -Plays an important role in immune function and protection –Take 10 000 IU per day

Zinc- One of the most important nutrients for the immune system -Take 50mg per day with food

Selenium- Works synergistically with Zinc and strengthens the immune system —Take 200mcg per day

Omega 3 Fatty Acids- Essential fatty acids work as immune enhancers, antioxidants and anti-inflammatories -Take 3000mg per day in divided doses

LIVER SUPPORT

LVDTX (Douglas Labs)- (*Contains Choline, L-methionine, Inositol, Betaine HCl, Lecithin, Niacin, Dandelion leaf, Turmeric, Milk thistle and Artichoke leaf*) —Take 3 tablets daily in divided doses with food

LCH (Thorne) (*Contains Dandelion root, Berberine, Stinging Nettle, Bearberry extract, Milk thistle and Burdock root*) —Take 3 capsules daily with food

SAT (Thorne) (*Contains Silybin Phytosome/Phosphatidylcholoine extract, Artichoke extract and Curcumin extract*) —Take 1 capsule one to two times daily with food

TAPS (Thorne) (*Contains Artichoke extract, Curcumin Phytosome, Picrorhiza, Silybin Phytosome*) —Take 1 capsule two to three times daily with food

NAC CystePlus (Thorne) (*Contains N-Acetyl-cysteine, a sulphur containing amino acid the precursor of glutathione which aids in liver support, detoxification and immune support*) —Take 1 capsule three times daily with food

Calcium D-glucarate (Thorne) (Contains Calcium D-Glucarate which has been shown to prevent the recycling of toxins while promoting liver detoxification) —Take 1 to 2 capsules three times daily with food

DIE OFF SUPPORTIVE NUTRIENTS

all recommended supplements are available online at www.drcobi.com

Psyllium -1/2 to 2 tsp of psyllium powder into 8 oz. of water (drink an additional 8oz of water to prevent constipation from occurring)

Medibulk (Thorne) *(Contains a Proprietary blend of Psyllium powder, prune powder and Apple pectin)* –Take 1 scoop in 8 ounces of water 1 to 3 times daily (drink an additional 8oz of water to prevent constipation from occurring)

Metafiber (Metagenics) (*Contains Rice bran, beet fiber, gluten-free oat fiber, apple fiber, cellulose, olive oil and d-alpha tocopheryl)* –Blend 1 level scoop into 8 ounces of water 1 to 3 times per day (drink an additional 8oz of water to prevent constipation from occurring)

Bentonite Clay- It is generally advisable to start with 1 tablespoon of bentonite clay daily, mixed with a small amount of water (Pay attention to the results for a week, and then gradually increase the dosage to no more than 4 tablespoons daily, in divided doses)

Molybdenum- Molybdenum is particularly useful during Candida Die-Off, when it helps your liver to expel the toxins that are produced when the Candida yeast is killed -Take 1000mcg 1 to 3 times daily.

Vitamin C- Buffered Ascorbic Acid powder is effective for individuals with sensitivity to the acidity of pure ascorbic acid -Take 2.5 grams up to bowel tolerance daily to help support the immune system

ADJUNCTIVE THERAPIES

SOFT HEAT INFRARED SAUNAS

Reducing toxic burdens of the body is a critically important factor in restoring health and vitality to individuals with chronic illness including Candida. The main drawback to using saunas in the past has been the discomfort many people experience during a sauna treatment. Traditional saunas use extremely high temperatures to warm the body by intensively heating the surface of the body only. Many people feel claustrophobic and find it hard to breathe. Fortunately, technological advances have resulted in a new type of sauna which is superior in many ways to traditional saunas. The new soft heat infrared sauna utilizes completely invisible infrared light to warm deeply inside the body tissues without heating the air or external parts of the body much at all. Many people who could not tolerate the traditional saunas will find the soft heat infrared sauna very pleasant and extremely effective at restoring health and well-being.

HEALTH BENEFITS INCLUDE:
- Weight loss (burn 600 calories in one half hour session)
- Pain relief from arthritis, back pain, chronic fatigue syndrome, fibromyalgia, headaches, etc.

- Eliminate harmful toxins including heavy metals, cholesterol, pesticides, environmental contaminants, etc.
- Increase circulation and cardiovascular function
- Clear cellulite
- Boost immune response
- Improve and eliminate skin conditions such as acne, eczema, psoriasis
- Recommended therapy- Thirty minute sessions taken 1 to 5 days per week as additional detoxification support as well sauna therapy aids in die-off reactions.

Epsom salts Baths (Avicenna)

Natural Source Epsom salt is extracted from an ancient underground deposit in Europe.

This natural Epsom salt is one of only a few natural deposits in the world and is recognized for its exceptional purity.

Epsom salt (magnesium sulfate) is reputed to aid in easing sore muscles and joints, restless leg syndrome and insomnia. Both magnesium and sulphates are absorbed through the skin and are vital to many body functions. Magnesium is an electrolyte critical to ensuring proper muscle, nerve and enzyme activity. Sulphates are needed for the formation of brain tissue, joint proteins and the walls of the digestive tract and are crucial for the generation of digestive enzymes.

Epsom salts assist in the elimination of metabolic compounds such as lactic and uric acid and helps to detoxify the body. It neutralizes static electricity build-up in our bodies from sources such as dry rooms, clothing and vehicles. It is a mild and gentle deodorant that does not disturb the skins natural balance.

Recommended therapy- Epsom salt baths are an excellent adjunct to any cleansing or detoxification program. Thirty minutes in a hot Epsom salt bath is recommended 1 to 4 times per week.

all recommended supplements are available online at www.drcobi.com

The following chart clearly summarizes the recommended supplements described previously.

Numbers 1, 2 and 3 consist of the basic fundamental treatment protocol. Numbers 4, 5, 6 and 7 include additional supportive nutrients that can be added to the fundamental protocol on an individual basis as needed.

	Month 1	Month 2	Month 3
1. Nutrition (additional detailed guidelines follow this chart)	No grains	0-1 cup Gluten free grains in their whole form only (NO GRAIN FLOURS)	0-1 cup Gluten free grains in their whole form only (NO GRAIN FLOURS)
2. Probiotics	Choose one: (to be taken throughout) - HMF Replete (first 7 days only) - Ultra Flora Balance - Sacro B - Multi Probiotic 4000 - HMF Replenish - HMF Intensive	Choose one: (to be taken throughout) - Ultra Flora Balance - Sacro B - Multi Probiotic 4000 - HMF Replenish - HMF Intensive	Choose one: (to be taken throughout) - Ultra Flora Balance - Sacro B - Multi Probiotic 4000 - HMF Replenish - HMF Intensive
3. Anti Fungals	Choose one and rotate each month: - Caprylex - Berbercap - Anti-MFP - Grapefruit Seed Extract - Yeast Balance Complex - Formula SF 722 - Candi Bactin AR - Candi Bactin BR - Oil of Oregano - Pleo Ex	Choose one and rotate each month: - Caprylex - Berbercap - Anti-MFP - Grapefruit Seed Extract - Yeast Balance Complex - Formula SF 722 - Candi Bactin AR - Candi Bactin BR - Oil of Oregano - Pleo Ex	Choose one and rotate each month: - Caprylex - Berbercap - Anti-MFP - Grapefruit Seed Extract - Yeast Balance Complex - Formula SF 722 - Candi Bactin AR - Candi Bactin BR - Oil of Oregano - Pleo Ex
4. Other Supportive Yeast Killers	Choose two: - Coconut oil - Colloidal Silver - Bentonite Clay - Psyllium Powder - Garlic	Choose two: - Coconut oil - Colloidal Silver - Bentonite Clay - Psyllium Powder - Garlic	Choose two: - Coconut oil - Colloidal Silver - Bentonite Clay - Psyllium Powder - Garlic
5. Die Off Support	As needed, usually only in Month 1: - Psyllium - Bentonite Clay - Medibulk - Metafiber - Molybdenum - HTC		
6. Immune Support	Choose two and take throughout or more: - Vitamin D3 - Vitamin A - Zinc - Selenium - Omega 3	Choose two and take throughout or more: - Vitamin D3 - Vitamin A - Zinc - Selenium - Omega 3	Choose two and take throughout or more: - Vitamin D3 - Vitamin A - Zinc - Selenium - Omega 3
7. Liver Support	Choose one: - LVDTX - LCH - SAT - TAPS - Cyste Plus - Calcium D Glucarate	Choose one: - LVDTX - LCH - SAT - TAPS - Cyste Plus - Calcium D Glucarate	Choose one: - LVDTX - LCH - SAT - TAPS - Cyste Plus - Calcium D Glucarate
8. Digestive Support	Choose one and take throughout: - BPP - Bio Gest - Dipan 9 - Ultrazyme - GI Digest	Choose one and take throughout: - BPP - Bio Gest - Dipan 9 - Ultrazyme - GI Digest	Choose one and take throughout: - BPP - Bio Gest - Dipan 9 - Ultrazyme - GI Digest

CANDIDA CONTROL DIET GUIDELINES

CATEGORY	TO INCLUDE	TO EXCLUDE
Fruits	2 servings (1 cup or 1 medium sized fruit) of domestic fruit only (berries, peaches, plums, apples, apricots, pears)	All dried fruits, juices and tropical fruits
Eggs, dairy, & dairy replacement	Eggs; plain unsweetened yogurt (cow, sheep, or goat) unsweetened coconut/almond milk, unaged goat cheese, Daiya cheese, Earth balance (butter alternative)	Cheese, butter, milk, sour cream, sweetened yogurt, butter, ice cream
Grains	None or Gluten free (brown rice, quinoa, tapioca, millet, buckwheat, amaranth, teff) **whole grains only. Only flours allowed**- coconut flour and almond meal	All refined or whole grains flours, breads, baked goods, products made with flour (except coconut/almond)
Animal Protein	Fish (fresh or canned) & other seafood, chicken, turkey, lean beef, lamb, (preferably organically-raised meats)	Cold cuts and all processed meats; Pork
Meat Replacements	Non- GMO tofu, tempeh	None
Beans	In small amounts, any dried beans, split peas, and legumes (not more than 1 cup (cooked)/day)	None
Nuts & seeds	Walnuts, hazelnuts, filberts pecans, almonds, cashews, flax seeds, pumpkin seeds, sunflower seeds, poppy seeds sesame seeds – whole or as nut butters	Peanuts and pistachios
Vegetables	Non-starchy vegetables – raw, steamed, sautéed, juiced, or baked (see shopping list)	Mushrooms and starchy vegetables: potatoes, corn, yams, sweet potatoes, parsnips, cooked beets
Fats and oils	**Coconut oil**, avocado, olives, cold pressed oils: olive, flax seed, sesame safflower, pumpkin sunflower, almond, walnut, organic canola	Margarine, shortening, processed oils, prepared salad dressings, spreads and sauces, mayonnaise
Acidic and fermented foods	Lemon and lime juices and vitamin C crystals as replacements for vinegar.	All vinegars and preserved foods: sauerkraut, pickles, other products preserved in brine or vinegar
Sweeteners	Stevia (herbal sweetener); Xylitol	All: sugar, white/brown sugars, honey, maple syrup, corn syrup, high fructose corn syrup, molasses, brown rice syrup, fruit sweeteners
Beverages	Filtered, spring, or distilled water (drink 8 cups per day), herbal tea, green tea	Soda pop, juice, alcohol, black tea, coffee, and non-dairy creamers

PLEASE READ ALL LABELS

Dietary Guidelines Explained

The following is included to help you understand the reasons behind the Candida Dietary Guidelines. In general, foods are restricted because of their carbohydrate (sugar) content. Additional foods are restricted as noted. These dietary modifications are usually implemented for 2-4 weeks to assess response to the program. Follow-up modifications are made on an individual basis.

- _Fruits and juice:_ contain the sugar fructose
- _Milk and milk products (cheese, cottage cheese, cream cheese, sour cream, etc.):_ contain the sugar lactose. (Yogurt, although a milk product, is virtually devoid of the milk sugar lactose and is thus acceptable unless you have a dairy allergy.)
- _Dairy substitutes: Most soy milks_ contain some type of sweetener, usually brown rice syrup.* Soy _yogurts_ contain various types of sugar (agave syrup, amazake, white grape juice concentrate, or honey). _Most soy cheeses_ contain maltodextrin* (see Sweetener) or modified food starch (see Grains). _Oat milk_ is made from oats (see Grains). _Rice cheese_ is made from a grain (see Grains).
- _Grains:_ although complex carbohydrates, they are broken down into simple sugars.
- _Beans and other legumes:_ high in protein, but also high in complex carbohydrates and are recommended only in small amounts (not to exceed 1 cup per day).
- _Peanuts:_ (high in the mold, aflatoxin) _and pistachios_: are moldy nuts which can exacerbate candida.
- _Starchy vegetables:_ broken down into simple sugars.
- _Mushrooms:_ from the fungi family and may cross react with candida.
- _Processed oils:_ "bad" fats and should be eliminated from any healthy diet.
- _Acidic and fermented foods:_ may provoke symptoms because of similarities to candida yeast or they may act as food for candida.
- _Sweeteners_: the favorite fuel source of candida.
- _Alcohol:_ a sugar and is a fuel source for candida.
- _Known food allergens:_ increase gastrointestinal permeability and further weaken the immune system. This results in a more hospitable environment for the candida yeast.

Foods that Eliminate Candida

Vegetables
- Artichoke
- Arugula
- Asparagus
- Bamboo Shoots
- Beet tops
- Bok choy
- Broccoli
- Brussels sprouts
- Cabbage – all types
- Carrots
- Cauliflower
- Celery
- Chives
- Cucumber
- Dandelion greens
- Eggplant
- Endive
- Garlic
- Green beans
- Jicama
- Kale
- Kohlrabi
- Leeks
- Lettuce – red or green leaf and all types of greens
- Okra
- Onions
- Parsley
- Peppers (all kinds)
- Radish
- Red leaf chicory
- Sea vegetables – seaweed,kelp, nori, dulse, hiziki
- Peas – all types
- Spinach
- Sprouts (broccoli and bean)
- Swiss chard
- Tomatoes
- Watercress
- Zucchini

Fruit (if tolerated)
(No more than 2 servings per day)
- Apples
- Peaches
- Pears
- Plums
- Blueberries
- Raspberries
- Blackberries
- Cranberries

Organic Meat and Fish
- Chicken, Cornish game
- Hens, turkey, duck
- Fresh wild ocean fish –
- Pacific salmon, halibut,
- Haddock, cod, sole,
- Pollack, tuna, mahi mahi, etc.
- Shellfish
- Water-packed canned tuna turkey, chicken, salmon
- Lamb
- Wild game (Buffalo, Venison, Elk)
- Lean beef
- Eggs

Meat Substitutes
- Non GMO Tofu
- Tempeh

Beans — 1 cup/day
- All beans
- Lentils – brown, green, red

- Split peas – yellow, green

All the above beans can be bought dried or canned without added sugar

OILS

- Coconut oil
- Almond
- Flax seed
- Organic Canola
- Extra Virgin Olive
- Pumpkin
- Safflower
- Sesame
- Sunflower
- Walnut

BEVERAGES

- Herbal tea (non-caffeinated)
- Mineral water
- Spring water
- Distilled water
- Green tea
- Rooibos tea
- Coffee alternative

DAIRY AND SUBSTITUTES

- Plain cow yogurt with live Cultures
- Plain goat yogurt
- Unsweetened coconut or almond milk
- Fresh, unaged goat cheese
- Daiya cheese

NUTS AND SEEDS

- Almonds
- Brazil nuts
- Chia seeds
- Cashews
- Flax seeds
- Hemp seeds
- Hazelnuts (Filberts)
- Macadamia nuts
- Pecans

- Pine nuts
- Poppy seeds
- Pumpkin seeds
- Sesame seeds
- Sunflower seeds
- Walnuts

All of the above can be consumed as nut butters and spreads (e.g. Tahini)

VINEGAR REPLACEMENTS

- Lemon and lime juice
- Vitamin C crystals

MISCELLANEOUS

- All spices
- Olives (without vinegar)
- Gluten free grains (brown rice, Quinoa, Millet,
- Amaranth, Buckwheat, Teff, gluten free oats, Tapioca)(only when tolerable)
- Braggs Liquid Aminos
- Coconut Liquid Aminos
- Coconut flour
- Almond meal
- Carob powder
- Lactic acid fermented
- Sauerkraut

Foods to Avoid:

Vegetables

- Corn
- Potatoes
- Yam
- Sweet Potatoes
- Parsnips
- Cooked beets
- Mushrooms

Fruits

- All tropical fruits
- Fruit juices
- Dried fruits
- Canned fruit
- Candied fruit

Nuts and Seeds

- Peanuts
- Pistachios
- Any roasted or salted nut

Meat and Fish

- Any smoked meat
- Any processed meat
- Any pickled meat
- Sausages
- Hot dogs
- Deli meats
- Pork
- Farmed fish

Beverages

- Fruit juices
- Soda pop
- Alcoholic beverages
- Coffee
- Black tea
- Energy drinks
- Coconut water

Sweeteners

- Artificial sweeteners
- Barley malt
- Brown sugar
- Coconut sap
- Corn syrup
- Granulated & powdered sugar
- Date sugar
- Dextrose
- Fructose
- Glucose
- Maple syrup
- Mannitol
- Molasses
- Monosaccharides
- Sorbitol
- Sucralose
- Sucrose
- Turbinado sugar

Grains and Seeds

- Wheat
- Cous Cous
- Bulgar wheat
- Semolina wheat
- Durham wheat
- Rye
- Kamut
- Barley
- Oats (unless GF)
- Spelt
- White rice

Dairy

- Butter
- Milk
- Cream
- Ice cream
- Sour cream

- Whipped cream
- Cow cheeses
- Whey

MISCELLANEOUS

- Yeast including:
- Bakers yeast
- Brewers yeast
- Nutritional yeast
- Yeast – leavened bakery products
- Yeast containing vitamins (look for those labeled "yeast free")
- Caffeine
- Edible fungi
- White vinegar
- Mustard
- Ketchup
- Worcestershire
- BBQ sauce
- Mayonnaise
- Maltodextrin
- Refined, cooked, hydrogenated, fractionated or superheated vegetable oils

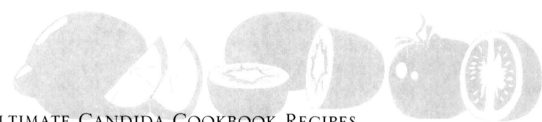

The Ultimate Candida Cookbook Recipes

Breakfast

Quinoa Porridge

1/2 cup quinoa, if not pre-washed make sure to rinse and drain before cooking
1 cup water
1/2 cup quinoa flakes
1/2 cup chopped domestic fruit (Apples, pears, peaches, berries)
Stevia or Xylitol to taste
1/4 cup chopped walnuts

Bring the quinoa to a boil, following cooking directions on package. Reduce the heat and simmer about 10 minutes, until cooked. Add the quinoa flakes, fruit, nuts and sweetener. Stir and continue simmering for another 10 to 15 minutes. The mixture should have a fluffy consistency.

Coco Cakes

4 eggs
1/4 cup coconut flour
1 pinch nutmeg
1 pinch cinnamon
Toppings (optional)
3 tsp. water
2 cups domestic fruit, mashed with a potato masher
2 tbsp. arrowroot
1/8 cup Stevia or Xylitol
1/4 tsp. cinnamon
1/4 cup coconut milk

Mix these ingredients and let them sit for five minutes. Melt coconut oil in your pan. Pour approx. 1/4 cup of batter for each crepe, allowing each side to brown before flipping it.

For the topping put the water, cinnamon, fruit, arrowroot sweetener in a saucepan and bring to a boil. Turn down the heat and simmer for 5 minutes until the sauce reduces and thickens.

CHIA BREAKFAST TAPIOCA

2 Tbsp. whole, white or grey chia seeds

1/2 cup of either almond or coconut milk (unsweetened)

Stevia to taste

Place chia in a small bowl and add the liquid. Stir well to try to submerge most of the seeds. Allow to sit 20-30 minutes, stirring once after about 5 minutes to prevent clumping. Stir again before serving. Makes one serving. Sprinkle a few blueberries on top and enjoy.

You can also mix the chia and liquid, cover and refrigerate overnight for a soft breakfast pudding the next morning.

ALMOND CAKES AND WAFFLES

1 cup fine almond flour

1/4 tsp. salt

1/4 tsp. baking soda

4 eggs

1 tbsp. Xylitol or Stevia equivalent

Coconut oil for cooking

In a bowl, mix the dry ingredients and set aside. In another bowl, whisk the eggs and add them to the dry mix. Adding more flour will thicken the mix, if desired. Spoon the batter onto a pre-heated waffle iron for waffles, or a frying pan/griddle for pancakes. Make sure to oil the surface of your cooking surface before adding the batter.

ALMOND CREPES

5 eggs

1/2 cup fine almond flour

2 tbsp. water

1 pinch salt

Coconut oil to cook with

In a large bowl, whisk all the ingredients well. Place batter in the fridge to thicken; approximately 10 to 15 minutes. After removing from fridge, be sure to stir before cooking. Use a crepe pan or shallow frying pan to make the crepes. These crepes can also be used as wraps for sandwiches.

BREAKFAST SAUSAGE

1/2 lb. ground turkey

1/2 cup very finely chopped onion

1 egg

1/2 tsp. sea salt

1/4 tsp. nutmeg

1/2 tsp. dried sage

3 tbsp. fresh chopped parsley

Mix everything together. Make into very small patties and fry in melted coconut oil until done.

SALMON OMELET

1/2 cup cooked wild salmon broken into pieces

1 tsp. olive oil

2 whisked eggs

1/4 cup chopped green onions

1 tbsp. non-fat plain Greek yogurt

Cayenne pepper to garnish

In a large non-stick skillet add the olive oil and heat. Pour in the whisked eggs so they cover the pan. Sprinkle the salmon pieces and green onions over the top. Allow to cook until the edges are done and then flip them. Continue cooking for another couple of minutes. Remove from pan and garnish with the yogurt and a dash of cayenne pepper.

GRAIN LESS SEED CAKES

1 cup raw pumpkin seeds

1-2 tbsp. whole anise seeds

2 tbsp. whole flax seeds

1/4 cup arrowroot

1 cup warm water

1 tbsp. oil

1/4 tsp. salt

1/4 cup water

In a large bowl, mix the pumpkin, anise, flax seed and arrowroot and mix well with a whisk. Take 1/2 cup of the mix and blend it in a blender on high for approximately 30 seconds. Using a spatula, move the mix from the bottom of the blender to prevent sticking and then continue blending for another 30 seconds. The mix should be very fine. Put it in a separate bowl and continue blending the rest of the mix in 1/2 cup portions until all the mix has been blended fine.

Don't clean the blender. Add the water, oil and salt and the ground mix and blend again. Pour the mix into a large bowl and let stand for 10 to 15 minutes. If you want to prepare this the evening before, you can let it rest overnight so it will be ready for breakfast the next day.

Use a non-stick frying pan and add a very small amount of oil to the pan and then spoon the mix into the pan. You can prepare a double batch and freeze them for later use.

SIMPLY MILLET MEAL

1/2 cup cooked millet

1 tbsp. ground flaxseed

1 tbsp. ground almonds

1/2 cup gluten free steel cut oats

Cinnamon

Coconut or Almond Milk

Stevia/Xylitol

Toppings:

Walnuts

Almonds

Pecans

Berries

Apples

Cinnamon

Mix the millet, flaxseed, almonds and oats together in a pot. Add in enough milk to make the mix moist and cook on low on the stove until thickened. Add in sweetener of choice and cinnamon. Top with toppings of choice and more milk, if desired.

GLUTEN FREE STEEL CUT OATS

Gluten free steel cut oats prepared as per package instructions

Toppings:

Walnuts

Almonds

Pecans

Berries

Apples

Cinnamon

Stevia/Xylitol

KINDA CAPPUCCINO

1 tsp. roasted chicory root

1 vanilla pod

1 cup unsweetened almond milk

Stevia or Xylitol to taste

In a sauce pan, add 1 cup of the almond milk and the seeds from a vanilla pod. Bring to a boil. Add 1 tsp. of chicory root and sweeten to taste.

BAKED GOODS

GRAIN LESS WRAP

3 tbsp. ground flaxseed

1/4 tsp. baking powder (aluminum free)

Pinch of sea salt

1 tbsp. melted coconut oil

3 tbsp. water

1 large egg or you can use 3 tbsp. boxed egg whites

Mix all the dry ingredients together and set aside. Mix all the wet ingredients together and pour into the dry ingredients. Melt a drop of coconut oil in a frying pan. Remove pan from heat. Pour in the batter and very gently work into the shape of a pancake. Once done, place the pan back on the stove and cook over low heat until you see the batter start to rise and get crisp along the edges. Gently turn and cook until done. You can make a larger batch and store in the fridge for a couple of days.

COCONUT BISCUIT BREAD

(This recipe has a consistency similar to corn bread or scones.)

3/4 cup coconut flour

1 cup shredded coconut

1/2 tsp. sea salt

2 tbsp. coconut oil (melted and slightly cooled)

Sweetener of choice, to taste (i.e. 1/2 tsp. Xylitol)

5 eggs

2 tbsp. coconut milk or unsweetened almond milk

1 tsp. aluminum free baking powder

In a medium bowl whisk the eggs and the melted coconut oil. Add the sweetener and salt and continue whisking. Slowly add the coconut milk/almond milk and continue whisking. In a separate bowl mix the flour, baking powder and shredded coconut.

Add the dry mixture to the liquid and stir with a wooden spoon. You will need to add more milk to get to the consistency of cake batter. Use a cake pan and line the bottom with parchment paper and grease the sides with coconut oil.

Pour the batter into the cake pan and drop the pan on the counter a few times to release any air bubbles and to even out the batter. Put into a 350 degree oven and bake for 30 to 35 minutes.

Place on cooking rack. Once cool, cover with plastic wrap and poke holes with a toothpick into the wrap. Place in fridge.

COCOROONS

4 large egg whites

1 1/2 cups unsweetened dried coconut

Sweetener of choice (i.e. 1 tbsp. Xylitol)

Vanilla bean (optional)

If you are using the vanilla, add it into the eggs, before you beat them. Beat the egg whites until they become firm and peak. Once the eggs are stiff, add the coconut and sweetener and very gentle fold in. Line a cookie sheet with parchment paper and, with a spoon, drop the mixture onto the cookie sheet. Bake at 350 degrees for 15 minutes. Remove from pan and place on rack to cool.

PUMPKIN SPICE IT UP COOKIES

2 cups almond flour

1/2 cup coconut flour

1 cup chopped walnuts

1/2 cup organic shredded coconut

2 tbsp. Xylitol or the equivalent of Stevia

2 tsp. cinnamon

1 tsp. allspice

1 tsp. ginger

1 tsp. nutmeg

1 tsp. baking soda

1 cup organic canned pumpkin

1/2 cup unsweetened almond milk

3 large eggs gently beaten

1 tbsp. grated lemon zest

Preheat oven to 375 degrees. Line a baking sheet with parchment paper.

Mix the coconut flour, almond flour, walnuts, dried coconut, sweetener, cinnamon, allspice, ginger, nutmeg and baking soda in a bowl and set aside.

In another bowl, use a whisk the blend the almond milk, canned pumpkin, eggs, and lemon zest. Add the wet mixture to the dry mixture and fold in until mixed. If the dough is too stiff, add a few splashes of the almond milk. The dough should not be stiff but easy to fold.

Use a spoon to drop the mix onto the prepared cookie sheet. Make sure the cookies are flat. Bake for 20-30 minutes or until the edges are browning. Let cool on cookie sheet then gently remove and place on a rack to continue cooling.

APPLE LOAF

2 cups almond flour or hazelnut flour

1 cup chopped walnuts

2 tbsp. ground flaxseed

1 tbsp. cinnamon

2 tsp. aluminum free baking powder

1/2 tsp sea salt

2 large eggs or Egg Substitute

1 cup unsweetened applesauce

2 tbsp. coconut oil

1/4 cup coconut milk

Preheat oven to 350 degrees. Coat a 9 x 5 inch loaf pan with coconut oil. Thoroughly mix the almond flour, walnuts, ground flaxseeds, cinnamon, baking powder and salt and set aside. In another bowl mix the eggs, applesauce, oil and coconut milk. Pour this mixture into the bowl with the dry ingredients and stir until combined. If the dough is too stiff, and a few drops of coconut milk to smooth it out. Press the dough into the pan and bake for approx. 60-70 minutes. Place on cooling rack.

SIMPLE MUFFIN MIX

2 1/2 cups almond flour

1/2 tsp. baking soda

1/2 tsp. salt

2 tsp. Xylitol or equivalent Stevia

3 eggs

1 cup fresh or frozen berries or chopped domestic fruit

Preheat oven to 300 degrees. Use baking cups to line a muffin tin. In a bowl, mix the dry ingredients and set aside. In another bowl, mix the eggs and sweetener and pour into the dry ingredients. Mix well. Add the fruit. Using a spoon, place the batter into the baking cups and place in the oven for 25 to 30 minutes. Cool on rack.

ALMOND BISCUITS

2 cups almond flour

3/4 tsp. salt

1 egg

1/2 cup melted coconut oil

Preheat oven to 325 degrees. Take a cookie sheet and line it with parchment paper. Mix the dry ingredients in a bowl and set aside. In another bowl, mix the eggs and melted coconut oil together. When you do this, be sure to whisk the eggs first and then gradually add the oil and you continue to whisk. Scoop 2 tbsp. worth of dough, roll into a ball and form into a patty. Place on the cookie sheet and continue until all the dough is used. Bake for 20 minutes. Store in fridge.

Cheesy Biscuits

3 cups almond flour

1 tsp. baking soda

1/2 tsp. salt

1/2 cup Daiya shredded cheddar

2 small onions, finely chopped

3 eggs

1 tsp. Xylitol or equivalent of Stevia

1/4 cup non-fat plain Greek yogurt

1/2 cup water

Preheat oven to 325 degrees. Line a cookie sheet with parchment paper. Mix the dry ingredients in a bowl and set aside. In another bowl whisk wet ingredients. Add the dry ingredients to the wet ingredients and mix well. Scoop approximately 1/3 of a cup of batter and put on cookie sheet and gently flatten so that each scoop is about 2 1/2 inches in thickness. Make sure to space well between each biscuit. Bake for 20 to 30 minutes, making sure that the tops are browned. Store in fridge.

Almond Flour Pizza Crust

1/2 cup almond flour

1/4 tsp. salt

1/2 tsp. dried basil

1/2 tsp. dried oregano

1/4 tsp. dried thyme

1 tsp. olive oil for cooking

Olive oil for preparing cooking surface

1 egg

Preheat oven to 325 degrees. Use parchment paper to cover the surface of a cookie sheet. Use olive oil to cover the entire surface of the parchment paper. In a large bowl, mix together the flour, salt, basil, oregano, thyme, olive oil and egg. This will create dough. Drop the dough onto the prepared parchment paper and spread it out thinly. Bake for 10 minutes. The dough should become firm and slightly browned. Use this crust as the base for any pizza you want to create. Remember, the consistency will not be the same as a regular crust pizza but it will provide you with a delicious alternative.

Flax Crust Pizza

6 tbsp. ground flaxseed

1/2 tsp. baking powder (aluminum free)

Pinch of sea salt

1 tsp. oregano

2 tbsp. melted coconut oil

6 tbsp. water

2 large eggs or you can use 6 tbsp. boxed egg whites

Mix all the dry ingredients together and set aside. Mix all the wet ingredients together and pour into the dry ingredients. Melt a drop of coconut oil in a non-stick frying pan. Remove pan from heat. Pour in the batter and very gently work into the shape of a pizza crust with even distribution. Once done, place pan back on the stove and cook over low heat until you see the batter start to rise and get crisp along the edges. The cooking process should take a while so that the top of the crust is not too sticky when you turn it over. Gently turn and cook until done. Once finished, let it cool and then place it in a 300 degree oven, on a cookie sheet. Bake for 10 minutes on one side and then turn and bake for another 10 minutes on the other side. The shape will reduce in size, but will become crisper. Let cool and then top as desired.

Marvelous Millet Crisps

1 cup millet flour

1/3 cup quinoa flour

1/4 tsp. baking soda

1/3 tsp. sea salt

Extra millet flour for kneading

1 tsp. arrowroot flour

Filtered water as needed (very small amount)

Preheat oven to 350 degrees. Mix all the dry ingredients together in a large bowl. Add the filtered water a little bit at a time, creating a dough consistency. Sprinkle some millet flour on a counter surface and place the dough in the middle. Start kneading; add a bit of millet flour as needed to keep it from sticking. Put the dough on a non-stick or coconut oil greased baking sheet and flatten with your hands to about 1/4 inch thick. Bake until browned and crispy. If you find that it is not as crisp as you would like, put back in the oven at 200 degrees for another 30 minutes.

Bean Meets Quinoa Crackers

1 cup mung bean flour

1/3 cup quinoa flour

1/4 tsp. baking soda

1/8 tsp. sea salt

1/4 cup millet flour for kneading

1 tbsp. arrowroot flour

1/2 tsp. of herbs of choice

Filtered water for kneading

Preheat oven to 350 degrees. Mix all the dry ingredients in a large mixing bowl and then add the filtered water a little at a time to create a bread dough consistency. Sprinkle some millet flour on a counter sur-face and place the dough in the middle. Start kneading, using more millet flour as required to keep from sticking. Put the dough on a non-stick or coconut oil greased baking sheet and flatten with your hands to about 1/4 inch thick. Bake until browned and crispy. If you find that it is not as crisp as you would like, put back in the oven at 200 degrees for another 30 minutes.

Eggless Coconut Bars

1/2 cup raw almond butter
1/4 tsp. vanilla liquid stevia
1/4 cup organic applesauce
1/4 cup coconut oil that has been melted
1 1/2 tbsp. ground flax seed
Mix all these ingredients together in a large bowl and then add the following:

1/4 tsp. salt
1/4 cup Xylitol
1/2 tsp. baking soda
1/2 tsp. xanthan gum
1/4 cup carob chips
1/4 cup shredded unsweetened coconut
2 tbsp. coconut flour
1 cup quinoa flakes

Mix everything together. Grease a square baking pan with coconut oil. Add the mixture and bake at 350 degrees for 15 minutes. Let it cool and cut into bars and keep in the refrigerator.

Eggless Lemon Bars

1 cup quinoa flakes
1/3 cup almond flour
1/3 cup shredded unsweetened coconut
1/4 cup melted coconut oil

Mix all of these ingredients together and pour into a square baking pan that has been greased with coconut oil. Make sure the mix is even across the pan.

In another bowl, mix:
1/2 cup coconut milk (the kind from the can!)
1/4 cup fresh squeezed lemon juice
1/4 cup Xylitol OR 8 drops liquid Stevia

Spoon this over the mix that is already in the baking pan. Sprinkle with 1/2 cup shredded unsweetened coconut and bake at 350 degrees for 20 minutes. Once cooled place in refrigerator for 6 to 8 hours, cut into bars and serve.

Eggless Walnut Chip Cookies
1/2 cup almond milk
1/4 tsp. xanthan gum
1 tbsp. ground flax
1/4 cup Xylitol

Put all of these ingredients in a large bowl. Using an electric beater, mix well and then add:
1/4 tsp. vanilla liquid stevia
1/4 tsp. sea salt
1 cup raw almond butter
1/4 cup coconut flour
1/2 cup quinoa flakes
1/2 tsp. baking soda
1/2 tsp. aluminum free baking powder
1/4 cup carob chips
1/2 cup chopped walnuts

Continue mixing with the electric beater. Spoon out the mix into medium size balls and place on a cookie sheet that has been lined with parchment paper. Flatten each ball so it is quite thin. Bake at 350 degrees for 20 minutes.

Raw Nut Balls
1/4 cup flax gel with seeds
Stevia or Xylitol to taste
1/2 cup raw almond butter
Unsweetened shredded coconut

Add sweetener of choice to flax gel. Add almond butter and continue mixing until totally incorporated. Roll the mixture into balls and roll the balls in the coconut making sure to cover the entire ball. Keep in the refrigerator.

Seedingly Nuttin Crust
3/4 cup Brazil or cashews
1/4 cup sesame seeds
1/4 cup tapioca or arrowroot starch
1/2 tsp. cinnamon (optional)
Pinch of salt
3 tbsp. boiling water

Preheat oven to 350 degrees. In small portions, grind the nuts in a blender and place in a bowl. Grind the sesame seeds and add to the ground nut mixture. Add the tapioca or arrowroot starch to the entire mix and blend well with a whisk. Add the boiling water and mix until it forms a ball.

Using unheated coconut oil, grease a pie plate and press the ball in the center. Making sure your fingers are wet, to prevent sticking, press the ball flat and work it evenly around the pie plate, as you would any pie crust. Place in preheated oven and cook for 20 minutes. Cool on rack.

ZUCCHINI MUFFINS

2 1/2 cups almond flour

1/3 cup coconut oil

1/4 cup yacon powder or syrup

3 cups grated zucchini

3 eggs, beaten

2 tsp. cinnamon

1/4 tsp. salt

1 tsp. baking soda

1/2 tsp. liquid stevia

In a large bowl, mix the flour, oil, yacon and zucchini. Then, add the eggs, cinnamon, salt, baking soda and stevia. Mix until well incorporated. Line muffin tins with baking cups and put in mixture. Bake in 350 degree oven for 30 minutes.

SOUPS

VEGGIE AND BLACK BEAN SOUP

2 tbsp. cold pressed extra virgin olive oil

2 medium onions chopped

1 small red bell pepper chopped

1/2 green bell pepper chopped

2 tbsp. minced fresh ginger

4 cloves minced garlic

1/4 tsp. red chili flakes

1/4 tsp. allspice

1/2 tsp. thyme

2 cans black beans that have been drained and rinsed

4 cups water

2 large cans of chopped tomatoes

1 cup celery cut into bite size pieces

1 tsp. salt

1 cup chopped cilantro

Black pepper

Use a large pot and heat the oil. Add the onions and cook until translucent. Then, add the peppers, celery, ginger, garlic, chili flakes, allspice and thyme. Cook for a few minutes until well blended and then add the black beans, water and canned tomatoes. Bring to a boil and then lower the heat and let simmer for 45 minutes to 1 hour. Add the salt, cilantro and pepper and serve. You can also drop a teaspoon of non-fat plain Greek yogurt to the top of each bowl.

CANNELLINI BEAN AND TOMATO SOUP

5 minced cloves of garlic
2 tbsp. cold pressed extra virgin olive oil
1 chopped large onion
1 chopped large leek
1 cup chopped carrots
2 cups water or chicken stock
1 28 oz. can of chopped tomatoes
1 tsp. rosemary
1 tsp. thyme
2 bay leaves
30 ounces cannellini beans
1/2 tsp. pepper
Salt to taste

Place the garlic with skins on and drizzled with 1 tbsp. oil into a 400 degree oven for 30 minutes. Peel and put aside. In a large pot heat the remaining olive oil, add the onion and leek, and sauté until translucent. Add the water (or broth), roasted garlic and can of tomatoes. Bring everything to a boil then reduce to a simmer and add the herbs. Continue simmering until the carrots are fork tender, remove from stove and let cool. Puree the soup mixture making sure to do this in small amounts. Put the pureed soup into another pot and add the beans. Put back on the stove and heat until the beans are cooked through. Season with salt and pepper.

VEGGIE STOCK

1 tbsp. cold pressed extra virgin olive oil
2 large onions chopped
2 stalks of celery chopped
1 red bell pepper chopped
1 leek chopped
4 large tomatoes chopped
6 cloves garlic, chopped
1 tbsp. dried parsley
8 whole peppercorns
3 quarts water

Heat the oil and sauté the onion, garlic, celery, pepper and leek and cook for about 5 minutes. Add the tomatoes, parsley, peppercorns and the water. Turn up the heat and bring to a boil and then turn down the heat and simmer for 3 to 4 hours. Strain the broth once through a sieve and a second time through a sieve that has been lined with cheese cloth. Let cool and freeze for future recipes or use right away.

Chicken Stock

Most of the store bought, prepared chicken stocks contain wheat, sugar or yeast so here is a recipe to help you create your own stock.

In a covered roasting pan, roast a small chicken, adding 1 large chopped onion and 1 large carrot that has been peeled and cut into big chunks. Pour in 1 1/2 cups of water. Sprinkle Braggs Amino Acid all over the chicken and then season with poultry seasoning and an assortment of spices of your choosing. Once the chicken has been fully roasted, remove the breast meat from the chicken for later use and put the rest of the carcass and remains of the roasting pan into a large stock pot. Add another large cut up onion, the leafy center portion of a celery heart and 3 bay leaves. Add enough water to just cover the contents and simmer for 4 to 5 hours. Let cool and then put through a large sieve. Once strained, layer the strainer with cheese cloth and strain again. You can freeze the stock in measured quantities to be used in a number of recipes.

Hearty Vegetable Soup

4 cloves of minced garlic
1 large onion, chopped
4 stalks of celery, chopped
1 small red bell pepper, chopped
1 cup cabbage, chopped
1 large zucchini, chopped
1 small crown of broccoli, chopped
1 tbsp. cold pressed extra virgin olive oil
½ cup tomato sauce
1 16 ounce can of tomatoes
4 cups vegetable broth (see recipe)
4 cups water
3 bay leaves
1 tsp. basil
1 tsp. thyme
½ tsp. pepper

Sauté all the vegetables in a large pot for 5 to 10 minutes. Add the can of tomatoes, water, veggie broth and tomato sauce and stir. Add the bay leaves and the rest of the herbs and cook on low heat for 2 hours.

VEGGIE CHICKPEA SOUP

2 cups celery, chopped

3 onions, chopped

2 cups zucchini, chopped

2 stalks of celery, chopped

4 tbsp. olive oil

2 quarts veggie stock

1 tsp. sea salt

1/2 lb. beet greens, chopped

1 cup cooked chickpeas

Chopped fresh parsley

In a large pot, sauté chopped veggies in oil until lightly cooked. Add stock and salt. Simmer at least one hour. During the last 15 minutes of cooking, add the chickpeas and beet greens. Garnish with parsley.

THAI COCONUT VEGETABLE SOUP

2 cups vegetable or chicken stock

1 can coconut milk

1 tsp crushed red chili flakes

6 to 8 cloves garlic, crushed

1 small onion, cut into half moons

1 red bell pepper, cut into strips

1 medium zucchini, cut in half lengthwise then sliced

2 cups thinly sliced bok choy leaves or cabbage leaves

½ cup chopped cilantro

Sea salt or Herbamare, to taste

Place the vegetable or chicken stock into 4 quart pot. Add the coconut milk, red chili flakes, crushed garlic, onion, and red bell pepper. Simmer for 15 minutes, covered, or until the vegetables are just tender.

Add the zucchini and simmer 5 minutes more. Remove pot from heat and add the sliced bok choy leaves, cilantro, and salt. Garnish with extra red chili flakes if desired.

ASPARAGUS SOUP

3.5 lbs fresh asparagus

3 large yellow onions, chopped

2 Tbsp. extra virgin olive oil

10 cups veggie stock

S & P to taste

Trim asparagus ends and chop into 1 inch pieces. Chop off the top 3 inches and set aside. Sauté onions in olive oil until soft. In a large pot, heat the stock, add the cooked onions and the 1 inch asparagus pieces. Simmer covered until the asparagus is soft.

Puree the soup in a food processor. Return it to the pot, season to taste and add the asparagus tops. Cook until the asparagus tops are just tender, about 5 minutes. Soup can be served hot or cold.

YELLOW SPLIT PEA DAL

2 teaspoons black or brown mustard seeds

A few tablespoons olive oil, coconut oil, or ghee

1 medium onion, chopped

1 tablespoon curry powder

Few pinches crushed red chili flakes

2 teaspoons grated fresh ginger

2 cups yellow split peas, rinsed well and drained

6 cups water

1 to 2 tablespoons tomato paste

Sea salt and freshly ground black pepper to taste

1/2 to 1 cup frozen peas

Chopped cilantro, for garnish

Heat a 4 to 6-quart pot over medium heat. Add mustard seeds and toast until they begin to pop. Quickly add the oil and onion and sauté until onion is very soft and beginning to change color, about 5 to 10 minutes. Then add the curry powder, chili flakes, and fresh ginger. Continue to sauté for another minute until you kitchen is very fragrant.

Then add the split peas and water. Bring to a boil, then reduce heat and simmer for about 45 minutes or until peas are soft and creamy. Wait to add the salt until the peas split.

LEMONY LENTIL SOUP

1 small onion, peeled

5 cloves garlic, peeled

2 tbsp. olive oil

2 cups red lentils

8 cups vegetable or chicken stock

5 cups baby spinach

Fresh parsley

1/2 cup fresh squeezed lemon juice

Sea salt to taste

Chop the onion and garlic in a food processor. Pour the oil into a large pot, heat and add the onion and garlic. Sauté until soft. Add the lentils and stock, simmer covered until the lentils are soft, approximately 30 minutes. Put the parsley and spinach in the food processor and mince. Add this mixture and the lemon juice to the pot of lentils and season to taste. Serve with a lemon wedge on the side. This can be ladled over cooked sprouted brown rice or quinoa (if tolerable).

Creamy Cauliflower Soup

2 tbsp. olive oil

1 chopped leek

2 crushed cloves of garlic

2 chopped stalks of celery

2 tsp. sea salt

1/4 tsp. white pepper

2 tsp. dried thyme

1 large head of cauliflower cut into chunks

6 cups water

1/2 cup raw cashews

1/4 cup chopped fresh tarragon

1/4 cup chopped fresh parsley

Add the oil to a large pot and sauté the leeks. Cook until soft. Add the garlic and celery and continue cooking until the celery becomes soft. Add the salt, pepper and thyme and stir. Add the cauliflower and mix until well incorporated and all the spices are evenly dispersed. Add the water making sure that it is enough to cover the cauliflower with a little extra on top. Once the cauliflower becomes soft add the tarragon and parsley. Using a measuring cup, remove 1 cup of the liquid from the pot and put it in a blender with the cashews. Blend on high. This will take on a creamy texture. Ladle some of the soup into the blender with the creamy mix and puree until smooth. Pour this mixture into a different pot and then continue to blend the rest of the mixture, placing the newly pureed mix into the new pot, until all the soup has been pureed. Add spices to taste and return to the stove. Cook on a low temperature until heated and then serve.

Slow Cook Turkey Rice Soup

1 lb. ground turkey

2 tbsp. olive oil

1/2 cup chopped onion

2 cloves of garlic chopped

3 stalks of celery cut up into small pieces

1 red bell pepper, cleaned and cut into small pieces

1, 28 oz. can chopped tomatoes

6 cups vegetable stock or chicken stock

2 tbsp. oregano

2 tbsp. basil

1 tsp. sea salt

1 tsp. pepper

1/4 cup fresh parsley

1 bay leaf

1 cup cooked sprouted brown rice

In a large skillet, brown the turkey and then drain off any fat. In a large pot heat the olive oil and sauté the onion and garlic. Put the cooked turkey, onions and garlic into a crock pot and add in the all of the rest of the ingredients, except the cooked rice. Cook on low for 6 hours. Add the cooked rice 20 minutes before serving.

LENTIL AND KALE SOUP

12 ounces of coarse chopped kale (about 1 bunch)

1 minced onion

3 minced cloves of garlic

1, 14 ounce can of diced tomatoes

1 minced stalk of celery

1 cup lentils

4 cups water

1 tsp. fresh minced jalapeno pepper (optional)

1/2 tsp. cumin powder

1/4 cup lemon juice

Put all ingredients in a large pot, except for the lemon juice. Boil and then turn down to a simmer. Continue cooking for 1 hour and then add the lemon juice.

CLEANSING CABBAGE SOUP

1/2 shallot, chopped

1 bunch scallions, chopped

1 leek, chopped

2 cloves garlic, minced

1 small zucchini, chopped

1/2 cucumber, chopped

1 small head of broccoli florets, chopped

1 cup green cabbage, shredded

1 cup Chinese cabbage, shredded

1 tomato, chopped

1 red pepper, chopped

1 fresh chili pepper, minced

4 cups vegetable or chicken stock

Salt and pepper to taste

Herbs of choice

After chopping all the vegetables, place them in a large stockpot and cover with stock of choice. Bring to a boil and then turn down to simmer. Simmer for 8–10 minutes. The vegetables should be crisp but cooked enough to be tender. Season to taste. This soup is very detoxifying.

CREAMY BROCCOLI SOUP

1 lb. fresh broccoli, chopped

1/2 of a cauliflower, chopped

4 cups vegetable or chicken stock

1 leek, chopped

2 cloves of garlic, crushed

1 stalk of celery, chopped

1 cup carrots, chopped

1 tsp. rosemary

1/2 tsp. thyme

1 bay leaf

1 tbsp. organic Herbamare

Salt and pepper to taste

Put all the ingredients in a large stock pot and cook until everything is tender. Once done, remove the bay leaf. Let the soup cool. Using a blender, blend the soup until smooth. Reheat and serve.

BURGER SOUP

1 lb. ground organic sirloin of bison

1 onion, chopped

2 garlic cloves, chopped

4 cups vegetable or chicken stock

1 tsp. thyme

1 tsp. basil

1 tbsp. parsley

2 cups water

1 cup carrots, shredded

1 cups shredded cabbage

In a large pot, fry the ground meat, onion and garlic. Once cooked, add the rest of the ingredients and bring to a boil. Reduce to a simmer and cook for 10 to 20 minutes and serve.

SAVORY BLACK BEAN SOUP

2 tsp. cumin seeds

1/2 tsp. chili flakes

2 tbsp. coconut oil

7 cloves of garlic, minced

1 large onion, chopped

1 cup black beans, soaked overnight and rinsed OR 1 can of black beans that has been rinsed

Water

2 tsp. turmeric powder

2 tsp. freshly grated ginger

In a large pot, melt the coconut oil and add the cumin seeds and the chili flakes. Sauté until golden. Add the garlic and onion and continue cooking until transparent. Next, add the beans and water. The amount of water you add will depend on how thick you want the soup to be. If using soaked beans, cook until tender. Finally, add the turmeric and ginger.

LENTIL SOUP WITH A KICK

1 small onion, chopped

2 stalks celery, chopped

2 tbsp. olive oil

1 tsp. chili powder

1 tsp. cumin powder

1 cup green or brown lentils that have been rinsed

4 cups vegetable or chicken stock

1 small can chopped tomatoes

1 small red or green pepper, chopped

1/2 cup chopped cilantro (optional)

2 garlic cloves, chopped fine

In a large pot, heat the oil and add the onion and celery. Cook until transparent. Add the spices and continue cooking another 5 minutes. Add the rest of the ingredients except for the peppers, cilantro and garlic. Continue cooking until the lentils are tender. Before serving, add the peppers, cilantro and garlic.

SNACKS AND SIDES

BABA GHANOUJ

2 medium peeled eggplants

1/4 cup sesame tahini

3 crushed cloves of garlic

1/4 cup chopped fresh parsley

2 tbsp. lemon juice

1/2 tsp. ground cumin

1 tsp. salt

Pepper to taste

1 tsp. olive oil

Preheat the oven to 400 degrees. Cut the stems off the eggplants and prick them all over with a fork. Put them in the oven, on the rack, and bake for 45 minutes until they are soft and wrinkled. Take them gently out of the oven and cool for a few minutes.

In a blender combine the tahini, garlic, parsley, lemon juice, cumin, salt and pepper in a blender and puree. Chop eggplant and add into blender and continue pureeing until the mixture is smooth. Remove from blender and drizzle with the oil and add pepper to taste.

Hummus

4 cloves of garlic, minced

1 tbsp. cold pressed extra virgin olive oil

1 can chickpeas, rinsed

4 tbsp. sesame tahini

3 tbsp. water

1 tsp. salt

1/4 cup lemon juice

1/2 tsp. pepper

2 tbsp. chopped fresh parsley (optional)

1/2 tsp. cumin

Add all ingredients to a food processor and blend until smooth.

If you don't want the garlic to have a strong taste, place the cloves, with the skins on, in a baking dish, drizzle with the olive oil and bake for 15 minutes at 400 degrees, or until soft. Cool and then remove the skins and add the garlic to a blender or food processor with the rest of the ingredients. Blend until smooth.

Veggie Dip

2 small tomatoes, finely chopped

2 medium roasted red bell peppers (see directions below for roasting)

2 large red onions finely chopped

3 minced garlic cloves

2 tsp. cold pressed extra virgin olive oil

1 tbsp. dried parsley

1 tbsp. dried basil

1 tbsp. lemon juice

Water as needed

Salt and pepper to taste

Put the tomatoes, whole peppers, onions and garlic (leave skin on garlic) on a cookie sheet. Drizzle with oil and roast in the oven at 400 degrees for 50 minutes, turning the veggies a couple of times during cooking. When they are done, the veggies should be browned and all the moisture gone.

Cool the veggies and then skin the peppers and remove the seeds and core and skin the garlic. Put everything into a blender or food processor and add the parsley, basil, and lemon juice. Puree until smooth. You may want to add water to help the process. Add salt and pepper to taste.

GUACAMOLE

2 avocados that have been peeled and mashed

1 large diced tomato

1/2 cup diced red bell pepper

3/4 cup finely chopped red onion

2 tbsp. lime juice

1/4 tsp. red chili flakes (less if you don't like hot)

1 clove minced garlic

1/4 cup chopped cilantro

Dash of ground cumin

Sat and pepper to taste

Mix everything together and enjoy!

KALE CHIPS

1 bunch kale

1 tablespoon olive oil

1 teaspoon seasoned salt

Preheat oven to 350 degrees. Line a cookie sheet with parchment paper. With a knife or kitchen shears carefully remove the leaves from the thick stems and tear into bite size pieces. Wash and thoroughly dry kale with a salad spinner. Drizzle kale with olive oil and sprinkle with seasoning salt. Bake until the edges brown but are not burnt, 10 to 15 minutes.

ROASTED CHICKPEAS

2 tablespoons olive oil

1 tablespoon ground cumin

1 teaspoon garlic powder

1/2 teaspoon chili powder

1 pinch sea salt

1 pinch ground black pepper

1 dash crushed red pepper

1 (15 ounce) can chickpeas, rinsed and drained

Preheat oven to 350 degrees. Whisk the oil, cumin, garlic powder, chili powder, sea salt, black pepper, and red pepper together in a small bowl. Add the chickpeas and toss to coat. Spread into a single layer on a baking sheet. Roast in the preheated oven, stirring occasionally, until nicely browned and slightly crispy, about 45 minutes.

VEGAN CHEESE

1 tsp coarsely chopped garlic

1/2 tsp sea salt

2 cups of raw almonds and cashews

1/4 cup fresh lemon juice

1/4 cup of water (as needed)

Place garlic and salt in a food processor and blend. Add nuts and process into small pieces. Add lemon juice and water. Process to mix well. Add more or less water to reach your desired consistency. Will keep 4 to 5 days in the fridge. Add fresh or dried herbs, olives, sundried tomatoes and/or turmeric for variety.

CHEESY SAUCE

This can be used to top any steamed vegetable.

1 tbsp. coconut oil

1 tbsp. coconut flour

1 cup unsweetened coconut milk

½-3/4 cup Daiya cheese

Melt the coconut oil on medium heat. Whisk in coconut flour. Once mixed, add in coconut milk and continue to whisk. Add Daiya cheese and continue to whisk until uniform and silky in consistency.

NOTE more Daiya cheese can be added for a thicker sauce

Optional spice ideas: turmeric, paprika, cumin, curry

FRESH CUT SALSA

1 cup fresh chopped tomatoes

1/2 cup finely chopped red onion or sweet onion

1/2 cup fresh chopped cilantro

1/4 tsp. ground cumin

1/4 tsp. salt (or to taste)

Fresh ground black pepper to taste

Mix all the ingredients together in a bowl.

LOVELY LENTILS

2 tsp. mustard seeds

4 tbsp. olive oil

1 onion, finely chopped

3 cloves garlic, minced

1 tbsp. peeled and grated ginger

1 tsp. ground turmeric

1 cup red lentils (soak overnight and remove the water)

4 cups water or chicken stock

1 1/4 cups coconut milk

Salt and pepper to taste

Heat the oil in a large frying pan and add the mustard seeds. Once the seeds are popped, add the onion and cook until translucent. Add the garlic and ginger in with the cooked onions and continue cooking for another 5 minutes. Sprinkle with the turmeric and mix thoroughly.

Add in the lentils, water or stock, coconut milk and salt and pepper to taste and continue to stir. Bring the mixture to a boil and then turn down the heat and cook for 1 hour.

SPANISH BROWN RICE

1/2 large red onion, finely chopped

1/2 large red bell pepper, finely chopped

1/4 large green bell pepper, finely chopped

2 cloves garlic, finely chopped

1 stalk of celery, finely chopped

1/2 tsp. cumin

1/4 tsp. oregano

1/4 tsp. black pepper

1/4 tsp. sea salt

1/2 cup diced tomatoes

1/2 cup tomato sauce

1/2 cup chicken or vegetable broth

1 tbsp. olive oil

2 cups cooked sprouted brown rice

In a large frying pan heat the oil. Add the onion, peppers, and celery. Cook for minutes or until the peppers are soft. Add the garlic and spices and cook for another 5 minutes. Add the cooked rice, tomatoes and tomato sauce. Stir well and add the broth of choice. Cook until moisture has evaporated and serve.

SPAGHETTI SQUASH PASTA

Cut the squash in half and use a spoon to clean out the seed portion. Drizzle inside of squash with olive oil; wrap each half in tin foil, place on a cookie sheet and bake at 375 degrees for 1 hour. Remove from oven and let cool. Once cooled, use a fork to scrape out the flesh which comes out in strands. Drain off any liquid and use just like spaghetti.

BASIC CHEESE

1 tsp coarsely chopped garlic (you can use less if you'd rather have a milder flavor)

1/2 tsp sea salt

2 cups of either almonds or raw cashews, or you can use 1 cup of each

1/4 cup fresh lemon juice

1/4 cup of water (as needed)

Place garlic and salt in food processor and blend. Add nuts and process into small pieces. Add lemon juice and water. Process to mix well. Add more or less water to reach your desired consistency.

Will keep 4 to 5 days in the fridge. Great as a topping for vegetables.

For variety, add fresh or dried herbs, olives, or sundried tomatoes.

TOMATO SAUCE

12 vine-ripened tomatoes

12 whole garlic cloves, peeled

Olive oil

Salt and pepper to taste

Preheat oven to 375 degrees. Make a small hole in the stem portion of the tomato and insert one garlic clove. Do this for each tomato. Rub the olive oil on the tomatoes and bake them on a cookie sheet covered in parchment paper until they are soft and cooked through. Once done, cool the tomatoes and then blend them in a food processor until smooth. Season with salt and pepper and store in the fridge for 5 days or you can divide into portions and freeze.

CELERY ROOT SMASH-UP

1 sweet onion

1/2 tsp. sea salt

1 tbsp. coconut oil

1 tbsp. olive oil

1 celery root

Salt and pepper to taste

Peel and cube the celery root. Put the celery cubes into a big pot with water and cook on high until tender. Drain the contents through a strainer and mash with a potato masher. Cover to keep warm and set aside.

Thinly slice onion, but do not mince. Place the coconut oil in a frying pan, add the onion and sprinkle with the salt. The salt will help bring out the natural juices of the onion and help with the cooking process. Cook the onion until it is browned and caramelized. If required, add a bit of water, should the pan become dry.

Take the mashed celery root and add the caramelized onions. Season to taste and serve warm. A great way to replace mashed potatoes.

BEANLESS HUMMUS

2 medium raw zucchini, chopped

1/4 cup olive oil

4 gloves of garlic, minced

2 tsp. sea salt

1/2 cup lemon juice

3/4 cup sesame seeds

1/4 tsp. cayenne

Put everything into the food processor and mix until smooth.

Cheesy Pumpkin Dip

Filtered water

2 cups raw organic pumpkin seeds

1 cup fresh parsley or cilantro, chopped

1 tbsp. minced garlic

1 tbsp. minced ginger

1 tbsp. minced jalapeno

1 1/2 tsp. sea salt

1/3 cup olive oil

1/2 cup lemon juice

Soak the pumpkin seeds in the filtered water for about 15 minutes. Drain in a colander and then put the soaked pumpkin seeds and the rest of the ingredients in a food processor and mix until smooth. Must be refrigerated.

Pesto

1/2 cup pine nuts

1/2 cup ground almonds

Handful of fresh basil

1 clove of garlic

Olive oil

1 tsp. lemon juice

Put everything into a food processor and drizzle in the olive oil to get a pesto consistency.

Mock French Fries

1 Celery Root

1 tbsp. Olive Oil

Sea Salt

Wash the celery root to remove any bits of dirt. Use a paring knife to remove the outer part. Cut the cleaned root into strips similar to the shape of a French fry. Place the cut pieces in a bowl and drizzle with olive oil. Toss to coat. Place the pieces on a cookie sheet lined with parchment paper making sure that they are well spaced. Bake at 375 degrees making sure to flip them a few times. You will know they are done when they start to brown.

Sesame Lentils

1 tsp. minced ginger

3 cloves of minced garlic

3 cups soaked lentils (alternatively a non BPA can of lentils can be used)

1 tsp. Bragg's Amino Acids

1 tbsp. sesame oil

1 tbsp. olive oil

Add the oils to a pot and then add the ginger and garlic and sauté. Add the Bragg's and the lentils. Continue cooking for another 10 to 15 minutes. Makes a great side dish.

Cheesy Cauliflower Mash

1 large cauliflower, chopped

1/2 cup cheddar Daiya, shredded

1 tbsp. Earth Balance

1 tsp. fresh, finely grated nutmeg

Salt and pepper to taste

Steam cauliflower until soft. Once cooked, mash the cauliflower and add the Earth Balance and Daiya cheese and until well incorporated. Add the nutmeg, salt and pepper and mix until incorporated.

Steak and Chicken Dry Rub Spice

2 tbsp. sea salt

2 tbsp. whole yellow mustard seed

2 tbsp. dried garlic flakes

1 tbsp. course ground black pepper

1 tbsp. coriander seeds

1 tsp. red pepper flakes

Put all the ingredients in a grinder or processor. Keep pulsing until well blended but not too fine. You want the mix to maintain some texture. Rub this mix on steak or chicken. Let it rest for 1/2 hour and then barbecue or broil in the oven. Store any leftover rub in a well-sealed jar.

Herb Salt

3 tbsp. dried cilantro

2 tbsp. dried basil

1 tbsp. dried dill

2 tsp. dried marjoram

1 tsp dried oregano

1/2 tsp. cayenne

4 tbsp. course sea salt

Put all these ingredients in a grinder or processor. Mix until fine. Put in a salt shaker and use to spice up your recipes.

No Fry Fries

1 jicama cut into fry shaped pieces

3 tbsp. olive oil

1/2 tsp. sea salt

1/4 tsp. dry garlic

1/4 tsp. cayenne

Dash of cumin

In a large bowl, mix all ingredients except for the jicama. Add the jicama and toss to coat. You're done! Enjoy.

Cauli Cakes

1 head of cauliflower, chopped

4 eggs

1 tbsp. chopped onions

Sea salt to taste

1 tsp. olive oil or coconut oil

Put everything into a food processor and mix until completely incorporated and fluffy. Form patties with the mixture. Add oil to frying pan and spoon on mix. Keep the portions small sized.

Cabbage with Dill

1 tbsp. coconut oil

1 head cabbage, chopped

1 onion, diced

½ tsp. celery seed

½ tsp. dill weed

Sea Salt to taste

Cayenne pepper to taste

In a large skillet melt the coconut oil. Add the cabbage and onion and cook until both items start to brown. Sprinkle with herbs and salt and serve.

Zucchini Roast

3 zucchini, cut into chunks

1 onion, sliced thin

Sea salt and pepper to taste

2 tbsp. olive oil

1 tsp. thyme

Preheat your oven to 450 degrees. In a large baking dish, place the zucchini, onions and thyme. Drizzle with the olive oil making sure everything is well coated. Place in the oven for 1/2 hour, making sure to flip the ingredients part way through the process.

Zucchini with Sesame

1 large zucchini cut diagonally
Tahini
Sesame Seeds
Sesame Oil

Preheat oven to 200 degrees. Line a cookie sheet with parchment paper. Place the sesame seeds in a shallow bowl. Cover one side of the sliced zucchini with the sesame oil and the other side the tahini. Place the tahini side of the zucchini in the sesame seeds and put the oil side down on the parchment paper. Bake for 20 minutes.

Coconut Milk Broccoli with Almonds

2 1/2 cup broccoli florets
1/2 cup coconut milk
2 tbsp. toasted almond slivers
Sea salt

Steam the broccoli until tender. Sprinkle with sea salt. Set aside. Put the coconut milk in a saucepan and cook until amount is reduced by half. Put the broccoli in a serving bowl, cover with the coconut milk reductions and almonds.

Garlicky Green Beans

1 tbsp. olive oil
2 large onions, chopped
6 cloves garlic, chopped
2 lbs. green beans, washed, tipped and cut in half
4 tomatoes, chopped
Water
Sea salt

In a large skillet, sauté the onions and garlic, until the onion is translucent. Add the green beans and cover with skillet lid so that they will cook in their own steam for approximately 1 minute. Add the tomatoes and water to cover the beans. Simmer until tender and add salt to taste.

Wild Rice Stuffing

1 cup raw, wild rice
1/4 cup Earth Balance
1/2 cup chopped almonds
2 stalks celery, chopped

1 medium onion, chopped

2 1/4 cups chicken broth

1 tsp. garlic powder

1/2 tsp. sage

Sea salt to taste

In a colander, rinse the wild rice with cold water. In a large, non-stick pot, melt the Earth Balance and add the almonds, celery and onion. Sauté until all the ingredients are tender. Pour in the broth and add the rice, garlic powder, sage and salt. Transfer everything to a large baking dish or casserole and cover with tin foil. Bake at 350 degrees for 1 hour.

Mexi Rice

1 cup long grain brown rice

1 tbsp. olive oil

1 1/2 cups chicken stock

1/2 onion, chopped

1/2 green bell pepper, chopped

1 fresh jalapeno pepper, chopped

1 tomato, chopped

Sea salt and pepper to taste

1/2 tsp. ground cumin

1/2 cup chopped fresh cilantro

1 clove garlic, chopped

Heat oil in a large pot and add rice. Cook for 5 minutes, constantly stirring. Add the chicken stock and bring to a boil. Add the rest of the ingredients, stir, cover and cook on low for 35-40 minutes, or until rice is tender.

Lime Infused Rice

3/4 cup slivered almonds

1 1/2 cups long grain brown rice

3 cups chicken stock

3/4 cup minced fresh parsley

1/2 cup scallions, finely chopped

1 tbsp. sesame oil

2 tbsp. fresh lime juice

Grated zest of 1 lime

Roast almonds in a frying pan on medium heat until brown and toasted. Put aside. In a medium sized pot, add the rice and stock. Stir until water boils, cover, reduce to low and cook for 45 minutes. Once cooked, leave cover on and set aside for 10 to 15 minutes to rest. Put the rice in a large serving bowl and add the rest of the ingredients, except for the almonds. Toss and garnish with the almonds.

Sautéed Lentils

1 piece minced ginger

3 cloves garlic

3 cups sprouted lentils

Dash of Bragg's Amino Acids

1 tbsp. sesame oil

1 tbsp. coconut oil

In a large pan, heat the oils and add the ginger and garlic and heat through. Add the lentils and Braggs' Amino Acids. Cook until the all the flavors have been absorbed.

Leeks and Spinach

1 leek, chopped

Spinach, sliced thin

1 tbsp. olive oil

Sea salt to taste

Steam spinach until tender. In a frying pan, heat the oil and add the leeks. Sauté until tender. Add the steamed spinach and salt to taste.

Garlicky Spinach

4 cloves garlic, minced

1 tbsp. olive oil

1/4 lb. cooked spinach

Fresh squeezed lemon juice

Sea salt to taste

2 tbsp. pine nuts

In a large frying pan, add the olive oil and garlic. Sauté for a couple of minutes then add the cooked spinach. Add some fresh lemon juice and sea salt. Top with pine nuts and serve.

Salads and Dressings

Hemp Seed Tabouleh

1 cup shelled hempseeds (you can find these at most health-food stores in the bulk section)

1 cup fresh parsley, finely chopped

1/2 cup fresh mint, finely chopped

1 cup cherry tomatoes, halved

1/2 cup black olives

1 cucumber, peeled and chopped

1 lemon, squeezed

1/2 cup olive oil

1/2 teaspoon sea salt

Mix all the ingredients together in a large bowl until combined. Chill for 30 minutes before serving. Enjoy!

Is that Really Tabouleh?

1 cauliflower, chopped

3 tbsp. olive oil

1 tsp. curry powder

2 bunches of parsley

Fresh mint (optional)

1 medium onion, chopped

1 large cucumber, chopped

1 large tomato, chopped

1/3 cup fresh lemon juice

1/4 tsp. salt

1/4 tsp. garlic powder

Place cut up cauliflower into a food processor and blend into granules that are even in size. In a non-stick frying pan, heat 1 tsp. of olive oil and curry powder so that it starts to cook but doesn't burn and stick. Add the prepared cauliflower and continue mixing and cooking for 10 minutes. Put cooked cauliflower in a large bowl and add some chopped mint, if desired. Then add the parsley, onion, cucumber and tomato. In another bowl mix the rest of the oil, lemon juice and salt with a whisk. Pour the dressing over the cauliflower mix and serve.

Apple Salad

1 cup cooked quinoa

1/2 cup chopped walnuts

1/2 small red bell pepper, chopped

1/3 cup red onion, chopped

1/2 cup fresh parsley, chopped

1/4 cup lemon juice

2–3 tbsp. vegetable broth

Salt and pepper to taste

1/4 tsp. cinnamon

1 clove minced garlic

1 large chopped apple

Make sure the quinoa is cooled, before starting this recipe. Mix everything together, except for the quinoa, walnuts and apple. Once mixed, add the quinoa, walnuts, and apple and incorporate.

WALDORF SALAD

2 stalks of celery cut into small cubes

1 medium apple, cored and skinned, cut into small cubes

½ cup chopped walnuts

½ cup raw goat cheese

In a large bowl, mix the celery, apple, walnuts and goat cheese so that the goat cheese crumbles and is well incorporated. Enjoy!

SESAME KALE SALAD

2 cups washed and chopped kale

3/4 cup carrots that have been julienned

1 small diced red onion

1 tsp. sesame seeds

Dressing:

1/2 cup Braggs Liquid Amino

1/8 cup sesame oil

1/2 tsp fresh grated ginger

Stevia or Xylitol for sweetness

Clean kale and remove large center stalk throughout the leaf. Chop. Place ice cubes and cold water in a large bowl and set aside. Bring a large pot of water to a boil and add kale. Cook kale for 5 minutes. Drain and put kale into ice water to stop the cooking process. Leave in ice water for 2 minutes then drain with a sieve. Once cooled, place in a large bowl and top with carrots and onion. In another bowl mix the Braggs, sesame oil, ginger and sweetener with a whisk. Pour dressing over the veggies, toss and serve. This mixture can also be used as the base for grilled fish or chicken.

BLACK BEAN AND AVOCADO SALAD

2 tbsp. lime juice

2 tbsp. olive oil

1/4 cup chopped cilantro leaves

1 jalapeno pepper, cored, seeded and chopped

1 clove minced garlic

1/2 tsp. salt

1 can black beans that have been drained and rinsed

1 1/2 cup thin sliced cucumber

1/2 cup diced red onion

2 avocados that have been pitted, peeled and diced

2 cups shredded lettuce

Put lime juice, olive oil, cilantro, jalapeno, garlic and salt in a blender and mix until well incorporated. Mix beans, cucumber and onion. Cover with dressing and mix well. Add avocado just before serving. Place shredded lettuce on a platter and spoon mixture on top.

Lentil Salad

1 cup sprouted cooked lentils

1 cup Romaine lettuce that has been ripped into small pieces

1/2 cup celery, very finely sliced

1/2 cup shredded carrot

1 large tomato, thinly sliced

Mix the lentils, lettuce, celery and carrot. Evenly arrange the sliced tomato on a platter and spoon the mixture over top. Drizzle with extra virgin olive oil and lemon juice.

Asian Slaw Salad

4 cups red and green cabbage shredded

Dressing:

1/4 cup fresh lime juice

3 tbsp. olive oil

1 tbsp. sesame oil

2 minced garlic cloves

1 tbsp. Bragg's Amino Acid

1 tsp. fresh grated ginger

1/4 tsp. dry mustard

1/4 tsp. cayenne pepper

Dash of Stevia or Xylitol

Mix all of the dressing ingredients together, whisk well. Pour over the cabbage and let it rest so that all the flavors marry well.

Chick Pea Salad

3 cups cooked chick peas

2 chopped purple onions

1/2 cup chopped black olives

1 chopped tomato

Dressing:

1/4 cup olive oil

1/4 cup fresh squeezed lemon juice

1 tsp. cumin

3 chopped cloves of garlic

Pinch of red pepper flakes

1/2 cup fresh chopped parsley

Mix the dressing together. Whisk well. Pour over the beans and let rest for 1 hour.

MOCK POTATO SALAD
1 head cauliflower, chopped
½ cup finely diced green onion
1 cup finely chopped celery
½ red bell pepper, finely chopped
½ cup finely cubed cucumber
Salt and pepper to taste
Dressing:
2 tsp. dry mustard powder
2 tbsp. lemon juice
1 cup Mock less Mayo (see recipe below)
2 hardboiled eggs, chopped
½ tsp. celery seeds
Paprika for garnish

Mix all ingredients and fold in dressing

MOCK LESS MAYO
1 egg
1/2 tsp. sea salt
1/2 tsp. dry mustard
2 tbsp. lemon juice
1 cup olive oil

Put egg, seasonings, lemon juice and 1/2 cup olive oil into blender or food processor and process on high speed. While blender is still running, remove the top to the small opening and slowly drizzle in the remaining oil. Continue until oil blends in and the mixture has the consistency of mayo. Store in refrigerator.

UNBELIEVABLE NO POTATO SALAD
3 large kohlrabi, peeled and diced
1 cup very finely chopped celery
1 medium onion very finely chopped
1 clove garlic finely minced
3 hardboiled eggs, chopped
1/2 cup mock mayo (see recipe)
1 tbsp. lemon juice
1 tbsp. dried dill
Sea salt to taste

Boil kohlrabi until tender. Do not let it get too soft! Drain through a colander and let sit until cooled. Add the rest of the ingredients, one at a time and mix.

Avocado and Bean Salad

2 tbsp. lime juice

2 tbsp. olive oil

1/4 cup chopped fresh cilantro

1/4 tsp. red chili flakes

1 finely minced clove of garlic

1/2 tsp. sea salt

¼ tsp. xylitol or stevia

1 can black beans that has been drained and rinsed

1 1/2 cups cucumber cut into small cubes

1/2 cup finely chopped red onion

2 avocados diced

Mix the lime juice, olive oil, cilantro, chili flakes, garlic, salt and sweetener and set aside. Gently toss the beans, cucumber, onion and avocados together. Pour the liquid mix over the top and gently mix again.

Tahini Salad Dressing

1 cup chopped celery stalks with leaves

1/4 cup chopped green bell pepper

1/2 of a medium onion, chopped

2 garlic cloves, minced

1/2 cup Braggs Liquid Amino's

3/4 cup tahini

1/2 cup lemon juice

3/4 cup olive oil

Put everything into a food processor and mix until creamy. Must be refrigerated.

Flax Dressing

1 tbsp. flax seeds

3 tbsp. lemon juice

4 tbsp. flax oil

2 tsp. dried dill

Mix the flax seeds in a food processor or coffee grinder. Once they are of a powder consistency put everything into a food processor and mix until smooth. Must be refrigerated.

Green Goddess Dressing

1 ripe avocado, chopped

1 minced clove of garlic

1 tbsp. lemon juice

1 tsp. chives

1 tsp. tarragon

Dash of sea salt

Put everything into a food processor and mix until smooth. Must be refrigerated.

Italian Dressing

1/4 cup olive oil

1/4 cup lemon juice

1/4 cup lime juice

1/4 cup unsweetened apple juice

1/2 tsp. oregano

1/2 tsp. dry mustard

1/2 tsp. onion powder

1/2 tsp. paprika

1/8 tsp. thyme

1/8 tsp. rosemary

Put all the ingredients in a blender and mix well. Keep in refrigerator.

Saucy Sesame

1 tsp. freshly grated ginger

1 tbsp. Braggs Liquid Amino's

1 tsp. sesame oil

1 tbsp. fresh squeezed lemon juice

1 tbsp. fresh sesame seeds

Put all the ingredients together in a bowl and whisk well. Excellent on fresh steamed veggies.

Coconut Dressing

1/2 can coconut milk

2 cloves of minced garlic

2 tsp. dill weed

Sea salt and pepper to taste

Whisk together and serve.

Basil Dressing

1/4 cup flax oil
1/4 cup water
3 tbsp. lemon juice
2 tbsp. fresh basil, finely chopped
1 tsp. minced garlic
Sea salt to taste

Put everything into a blender, mix well, and serve.

Main Event

Tofu Scramble

1 tbsp. coconut oil
1/2 chopped small red onion
2 cloves of minced garlic
1/2 sliced medium size zucchini
1/2 chopped red bell pepper
1/2 pound firm non-GMO organic tofu that has been drained and chopped
1/4 tsp. dried rosemary and/or basil
Salt and pepper to taste

Heat the oil in a frying pan and add the onion, garlic, zucchini and pepper. Cook until the vegetables are softened. Add the tofu to the vegetables in the frying pan and cook for 2 minutes until done. Add the herbs and cook until they are heated and incorporated.

Hearty Bean Stew

1 large yellow bell pepper
1 large red bell pepper
4 cloves garlic roasted
2 tbsp. cold pressed extra virgin olive oil
1 large onion sliced
1, 16 oz. can of diced tomatoes
½ small zucchini cut into bite size pieces
2 cups vegetable or chicken stock
1, 28 oz. can cannellini beans that have been washed and drained
2 tbsp. chopped parsley
½ tsp. dried rosemary
1 tbsp. lemon juice
½ tsp. pepper

In a 400 degree oven roast the peppers and unpeeled garlic that have been drizzled with oil. Roast for 30 minutes and put aside until cooled.

In a large pot heat the oil and add the onion and zucchini and cook for about 5 minutes. Add the stock of choice and boil. Add the beans, can of diced tomatoes, parsley and rosemary and continue cooking for about 15 minutes. Take the peppers and remove the skins and the core. Take the garlic and remove the skin. Chop both of these ingredients and add to the soup along with the lemon juice. Continue cooking until well mixed and heated throughout. Add pepper to taste.

COCONUT VEGETABLE CURRY WITH CHICKPEAS

2 tbsp. virgin coconut oil or extra virgin olive oil

1 tbsp. finely chopped fresh ginger

1 ½ tsp cumin seeds

2 cups diced celery

½ tsp turmeric

2 tsp coriander

1 tsp curry powder

1 tbsp. tomato paste

1 can coconut milk

¼ to ½ cup water

2 small zucchini, diced

2 cups cooked chickpeas (garbanzo beans)

2 tsp sea salt

½ cup cilantro

In a large pot, heat olive oil over medium heat. Add ginger, cumin seeds and cook for 1 to 2 minutes, or until the seeds begin to "pop". Add celery, turmeric, coriander, and curry powder. Stir well and continue to cook for another minute or so. Add the tomato paste, coconut milk, water and stir well. Simmer, covered, for 5 to 10 minutes carrots are almost done but still a little crisp. Add zucchini, chickpeas, and sea salt. Cover the pot and simmer until vegetables are tender, about another 6 to 7 minutes. Remove from heat and stir in chopped cilantro.

CURRIED GARBANZO BEAN AND ZUCCHINI STEW

2 tbsp. virgin coconut oil or extra virgin olive oil

1 medium onion, chopped

4 to 5 cloves garlic, crushed

2 tsp curry powder

1 tsp ground cumin

1 tsp ground coriander

½ tsp turmeric

½ tsp cinnamon

Pinch cayenne pepper

2 cups diced zucchini

2 cups diced tomatoes, or one 14 ounce can

3 to 4 cups chopped kale or spinach

3 cups cooked garbanzo beans, or 2 cans

1 cup bean cooking liquid or water

1 to 2 tsp sea salt or Herbamare

Heat an 11 inch skillet or 6 quart pot over medium heat. Add coconut oil, then onions. Sauté for about 15 minutes or until soft. Then add the crushed garlic and spices, sauté for a minute more. Next add the zucchini and tomatoes. Place lid on the pot and simmer over low to medium-low heat until zucchini is tender, about 10 minutes. Then add the chopped kale, cooked garbanzo beans, bean cooking liquid, and sea salt. Gently stir together and simmer for an additional 5 minutes. Taste and add more salt and seasoning if desired.

VEGETABLE JALFREZI

1 medium onion, chopped

2 inch piece of fresh root ginger, peel and finely slice

2 cloves garlic, finely chopped

1 small bunch of cilantro, chopped

2 red bell peppers, roughly chopped

1 cauliflower, broken into florets

3 ripe tomatoes, quartered

1 small butternut squash, peeled, cleaned and sliced into 1 inch wedges

1 15 oz. can of garbanzo beans, drained

2 tbsp. olive oil

1/2 cup Jalfrezi or medium curry paste

2 14 oz. cans of diced tomatoes

1 lemon

Heat a large pot on medium high heat and add 2 tbsp. olive oil. Add the onions, ginger, garlic and cilantro until golden, about 10 minutes. Add the peppers, squash, beans and Jalfrezi paste. Stir to coat. Add the cauliflower and fresh and canned tomatoes. Pour 1 1/2 cups water into pan, stir again and bring to a boil. Cover, reduce heat and simmer for about 45 minutes. If there is too much liquid, leave lid off for the last 15 minutes. Salt and pepper to taste and squeeze lemon on top.

GINGER CHICKEN STIR-FRY

12 oz. boneless, skinless chicken breasts, cut into bite sized pieces

1 tbsp. extra virgin olive oil

1 clove garlic, minced

1 tbsp. fresh ginger, chopped

1 onion, cut into wedges

Red bell pepper, cut into strips

1 cup broccoli, cut into bite sized pieces

1/2 c chicken stock, divided

1 tsp arrowroot powder

2 Tbsp. Bragg's Amino Acid

Heat oil in large skillet or wok and add chicken. Cook for approximately 5 minutes. Remove and set aside. Add garlic, ginger, onion, peppers, broccoli and 1/4 cup chicken stock to the skillet. Sauté for 5 minutes. Meanwhile, mix the arrowroot powder into the remaining 1/4 cup chicken stock and Bragg's Amino Acids. Return chicken to skillet, add Bragg's mixture and boil. Stir until the sauce thickens.

TURKEY TACOS

1/2 onion, diced

2 celery stalks, diced

2 tbsp. extra virgin olive oil

1 lb. ground turkey

1 clove garlic, minced

1/2 can tomato paste

1 tbsp. chili powder

1/2 tsp. cumin

1/4 cup cilantro, chopped

Whole lettuce leaves

1/2 cup fresh salsa

1/2 cup non-fat Greek yogurt

Daiya cheese, shredded (optional)

Heat the olive oil in a large skillet and sauté the onion and celery until soft, about 8 -10 minutes. Crumble the ground turkey into the skillet and add the garlic. Cook until turkey is browned. Stir in the tomato paste, chilli powder, cumin and 1/2 cup of water. Simmer for about 10-15 minutes. Add cilantro and season with sea salt and pepper to taste.

Scoop desired amount of turkey mixture onto lettuce leaf and add yogurt and cheese.

HALIBUT WITH LEEKS

2 leeks, white parts, sliced

4 halibut fillets, 1 inch thick; skin removed

4 tbsp. extra virgin olive oil

1/2 cup fresh oregano, chopped

Preheat oven to 375. Make 4 parchment squares. Place the leeks in the center of each square. Place the halibut on top of the leeks. Drizzle with the olive oil, and sprinkle with Oregano. Season with salt and pepper. Fold the parchment over several times to seal. Place a single layer on a baking sheet. Bake for 25 minutes. Remove from the oven, and transfer each packet to a plate.

Salmon Parcels

2 cups green beans, trimmed

3 lemons

4 salmon fillets, skin on

1 tbsp. extra virgin olive oil

Preheat oven to 400. Cut 4 sheets of aluminum foil for each fillet of salmon. Put a handful of beans in the middle of each piece of foil and lay a salmon fillet on top, drizzle with olive oil, squeeze half of a lemon over the top and season with salt and pepper. Fold up aluminum foil to seal the packets and place on a baking sheet. Cook for 15 minutes. Remove from oven and serve with lemon wedges.

Zucchini Lasagna

1 pound free range extra lean ground beef

1 large onion finely chopped

3 cloves of garlic, minced

1 red finely chopped

1 jar of organic spaghetti sauce

3 tablespoons organic tomato paste

2 bay leaves

1 tsp oregano

1 tsp basil

2 tablespoon coconut oil

No Salt Seasoning (yeast free)

1 tablespoon Braggs Amino Acids

Daiya cheddar cheese, shredded

2 large zucchini sliced lengthwise into thin, wide strips

9" x 12" glass lasagna pan

In a large pot, pour a small amount of warm water. Add the ground beef and work it into the water. Allow to simmer, and continue stirring, until the beef is cooked. Drain off all excess liquid and reserve the ground beef for later.

Melt 2 tablespoons coconut oil in pot and add the onion, garlic and red pepper. Sauté until soft. Add the reserved, cooked ground beef and spaghetti sauce and continue stirring. Add the 3 tablespoons of tomato paste and incorporate until well blended. Add the bay leaf and spices. Simmer for 1 hour and then cool. Once cool, remove the bay leaves.

Place the thin slices of zucchini across the bottom of the lasagna pan. Add 3/4 of the meat sauce to the top of the slices, making sure to cover evenly. Add more thin slices of zucchini as the next layer, making sure to cover completely, and then evenly add the remaining meat sauce. Cover the entire top with the shredded cheese. Bake, uncovered, at 350 degrees for 1 hour. Let cool for 5 minutes and serve.

Broccoli, Cheese and Chicken Bake

2 free range chicken breast halves cut into small pieces

2 tbsp. coconut oil

4 medium tomatoes, chopped

5 cups broccoli, chopped

4 medium green onions, chopped

1/2 cup cooked quinoa

1/2 cup Daiya cheddar cheese (shredded)

No salt seasoning (without yeast) to taste

Red chili flakes to taste

Sea salt to taste

Pepper to taste

1 tsp. paprika

1 tsp. oregano

1 tsp. basil

9" x 12" glass lasagna pan

In large pot, melt the coconut oil. Add the chicken pieces and cook for about 2 minutes. Add the green onions and tomatoes and cook until the tomato juices are present. Add the broccoli and continue cooking for 3 minutes. Add the quinoa and spices and mix thoroughly.

Pour the mixture evenly into a lasagna pan and sprinkle with the Daiya cheese and bake at 350 degrees for 1/2 hour.

Turkey and Zucchini Casserole

1 tbsp. olive oil

1 pound ground turkey

3/4 cup red onion, chopped finely

2 cloves garlic, minced

2, 10 ounce package of chopped, frozen spinach (squeeze out all the excess fluid)

1/2 tsp. basil

1/4 tsp. grated nutmeg

2/3 cup water

1–2 tsp. arrowroot

1/2 Daiya mozzarella cheese, shredded

2 small zucchini, thinly sliced

Salt and pepper, to taste

Preheat oven to 350 degrees. Then, in a large frying pan heat the oil and brown the ground turkey along with the onion and garlic. Once cooked, make sure to remove all the excess fat and then add the spinach, basil and nutmeg. Make sure to incorporate all the ingredients well. Mix arrowroot and water in a separate bowl and pour over mixture and combine.

Transfer the mixture into an 11 x 17 inch casserole dish and evenly arrange over the top. Sprinkle with the Daiya cheese and season with salt and pepper. Cover casserole with tin foil and bake in preheated oven for 30 minutes. After 30 minutes, take off the tin foil and bake for another 10 minutes.

CURRY-UP CHICKEN

1/2 tsp. ground cardamom
1/2 tsp. ground cinnamon
1/4 tsp. ground cloves
1/2 tsp. ground coriander
1/2 tsp. cumin
1/2 tsp. sea salt and fresh ground pepper
1/4 tsp. ground turmeric
1/2 tsp. chili powder
4 skinless, boneless chicken breasts cut into cubes
1 tbsp. olive oil
1 large red onion, chopped
6 cloves of garlic, minced
1 small red bell pepper, sliced
1/2 small zucchini, sliced
1 small tomato, chopped
3 tsp. arrowroot
14 ounces coconut milk
1 tbsp. ginger, peeled and minced

Mix the cardamom, cinnamon, cloves, coriander, cumin, salt, pepper, turmeric, and chili power in a large bowl and set aside. Add the cubed chicken breast pieces, mix through and set aside for 30 minutes.

Using a large frying pan, heat the oil and sauté the onion, garlic, red bell pepper, tomato and zucchini. Cook for 5 minutes and then place the ingredients in a bowl.

Add a bit more oil to the pan and put the chicken breast mixture into the already used pan and cook the chicken until tender. Once done, put the chicken into the bowl with the cooked vegetables.

In another bowl, mix the arrowroot and coconut milk until well incorporated. Pour this mixture into the pan that was used and cook until thickened. Add the ginger, cooked chicken and vegetables, cook for another 10 minutes and serve.

STUFFED PEPPERS

4 large red bell peppers

3/4 cup cooked quinoa

2 tsp. olive oil

Olive oil to drizzle on peppers

1 cup red onion, chopped fine

1/2 tsp. ground cumin

1/4 cup chopped cilantro

1 tbsp. lime juice

1/2 cup pine nuts

Salt to taste

1/2 tsp. ground pepper

Preheat your oven to 450 degrees. Wash and clean out the peppers, making sure to remove all the seeds and core, and then cut the peppers in half. Line a baking dish with parchment paper, place the cut peppers on the parchment paper cut-side down and drizzle with olive oil. Bake until tender, approximately 10 to 15 minutes. Remove pan from oven and turn the heat down to 350 degrees.

In a large frying pan cook the onions in the olive oil, until translucent. Add the cumin and cook until onions have been well incorporated with the spice. Then, add the cilantro, lime juice, cooked quinoa and pine nuts. Mix well and season to taste. Place this mixture into each of the cooked pepper halves and bake at 350 degrees for 20 minutes.

ITALIAN CHICKEN

1 tbsp. olive oil

2 boneless skinless chicken breasts cut into bite sized pieces

1 large onion, finely chopped

1/2 red bell pepper, chopped

3 cloves of garlic, minced

1 small zucchini, cut into pieces

1 small leek, chopped

1 14 ounce can of stewed tomatoes

1 cup tomato sauce

1 tsp. rosemary

1/2 tsp. salt

Pepper to taste

Heat the oil in a Dutch oven and add the chicken. Cook until browned and place cooked chicken in a bowl. Add the onion, pepper, garlic, zucchini and leek to the pan and cook for 15 minutes. Incorporate the tomatoes and tomato juice and add the cooked chicken and rosemary. Cover and simmer for 20 minutes. Season to taste.

VEGGIE LOAF

2 tbsp. olive oil

1 large onion, chopped

1 tbsp. arrowroot

1 tsp. thyme

3/4 cup water

1 cup walnuts, chopped fine

1 cup cashews, chopped fine

1 cup quinoa puffs

1 tbsp. lemon juice

1/2 tsp. salt

1/4 tsp. fresh ground pepper

2 cloves garlic, minced

Preheat oven to 400 degrees. In a large pan, add the oil and cook the onions for about 5 minutes and then add the garlic and cook for another 2 minutes. Add the arrowroot, thyme, water and cook until thickened. Then add the nuts and quinoa puffs. Remove from heat and add the lemon juice and season to taste. Blend everything until well moistened.

Grease a loaf pan and add the mixture, making sure to press mixture to make it uniform. Put into the oven and bake for 30 minutes. Remove and slice.

MEXICAN CHICKEN

1 cup salsa (see recipe)

1/4 cup water

2 cloves minced garlic

1 tbsp. olive oil

4 skinless, boneless chicken breasts

Salt and pepper to taste

In a frying pan, on very low temperature, heat the oil and sauté the garlic for about 1 minute. Place the chicken breasts in the pan. Cook each side for 5 minutes. Top the chicken breasts with the salsa, season with salt and pepper and cover. Simmer for 30 minutes, until done.

CHILI CON-QUINOA

1 cup cooked quinoa

1 large onion, chopped

1 large green bell pepper, finely chopped

1 large red bell pepper, finely chopped

1 tsp. red chilli flakes (less or omit, if you don't like too much heat)

1 14 ounce can of black beans that have been rinsed

1, 28 ounce can of crushed tomatoes

1 tbsp. chili powder

1 tsp. oregano

2 tsp. cumin

Salt and pepper to taste

In a large frying pan heat the oil and add the onion and bell peppers. Cook for 10 minutes. Add the beans, crushed tomatoes, herbs and spices. Cook on low for 30 minutes and then add the quinoa until heated through. Season to taste. You can also add a drop of non-fat plain Greek yogurt to the top of each bowl served.

ZUCCHINI BURGERS

1 1/2 cups grated zucchini

2 cloves of minced garlic

1/2 small onion, finely chopped

1 egg

2 tbsp. olive oil

1 tsp. basil

1 tsp. oregano

1/2 tsp. parsley

1 cup garbanzo bean flour

Salt and pepper to taste

Coconut oil for frying

Place the chopped vegetables in a large bowl and add the egg, olive oil, herbs, flour, salt and pepper. Mix well.

Heat the coconut oil in a large frying pan and spoon drop the mixture forming patties that are about 1/2 inch thick. On medium heat cook until they are browned on both sides, about 5-7 minutes per side.

LENTIL PATTIES

3/4 cup pink lentils that have been soaked overnight

3 tbsp. vegetable stock (may require more)

3 cups chopped, fresh spinach

2 tbsp. finely chopped green onions

1 clove minced garlic

1/2 tsp. salt

1 tbsp. chopped cilantro

2 tsp. arrowroot flour

3 tbsp. coconut oil

Drain the lentils and puree with vegetable stock. Pour mix into a large bowl. Keep the coconut oil aside for frying. Add the rest of the ingredients and mix thoroughly.

In a large frying pan heat the coconut oil until melted. Spoon drop the mixture into the frying pan and press into patties. Each side will take about 2 minutes to cook. They should be browned on both sides.

FRITTATA

1 cup Daiya shredded cheddar cheese

1/4 cup almond flour

1/4 cup Italian parsley

1 tbsp. olive oil

2 onions, finely chopped

2 garlic cloves, minced

1 green bell pepper, sliced

1 red bell pepper, sliced

5 eggs, beaten

1/2 cup non-fat plain Greek yogurt

1 tsp. salt

Preheat oven to 350 degrees. In a large bowl, mix the Daiya cheese, almond flour, parsley and set aside. Heat the olive oil in a frying pan and sauté the onions and garlic on low heat. Add the peppers and sauté until any liquids are evaporated. In another bowl, mix the beaten eggs, yogurt and salt and then transfer the liquid mix to the bowl with the dry mix and add the contents of the frying pan. Combine well. Pour into an 8 inch square casserole dish and bake for 40 to 50 minutes. The frittata should be nicely browned, on top. Once done, let it cool before cutting into portions.

EASY TUNA SALAD

2 6 oz. cans of tuna packed in water

1 tomato that has been diced

1 red bell pepper that has been diced

1 large cucumber that has been diced

1/2 cup chopped fresh dill

2 tbsp. fresh squeezed lemon juice

Salt and pepper to taste

Place drained tuna in a large bowl and break it up. Add the rest of the ingredients and mix well. For a spicier tuna salad, add 1/4 tsp of red chili flakes.

This can be made into a tuna melt (See following Tuna Melt recipe)

TUNA MELT

1/2 cup almond flour

1/4 tsp. salt

1/2 tsp. dried basil

1/2 tsp. dried oregano

1/4 tsp. dried thyme

1 tsp. olive oil for cooking

Olive oil for preparing cooking surface

1 egg

Easy Tuna Salad (see recipe)

1/2 cup Daiya cheddar cheese shredded

Preheat oven to 325 degrees. Use parchment paper to cover the surface of a cookie sheet. Use olive oil to cover the surface of parchment paper. In a large bowl, mix together the flour, salt, basil, oregano, thyme, olive oil and egg. This will create dough. Drop the dough onto the prepared parchment paper and spread it out thinly. Bake for 10 minutes. The dough should become firm and slightly browned. Remove from oven and place the Easy Tuna Salad mix on top and sprinkle with the Daiya cheese. Put back in the oven for another 5 minutes. This can be eaten right after baking.

SAVOURY ZUCCHINI PANCAKES

2 cups of grated zucchini

1 small finely chopped onion

1 minced clove of garlic

1 egg

2 tbsp. almond flour

Salt and pepper to taste

1 tsp. coconut oil

Mix everything together to form a batter. You may need to adjust the amount of almond flour, depending on the moisture content of the zucchini. The batter should adhere to a spoon but not be runny. Melt coconut oil in a frying pan and place spoonfuls of the mixture onto the surface and then flatten with the spatula. Cook on both sides until brown. You can serve these with a topping of fresh salsa and non-fat plain Greek yogurt.

CHICKEN CHILI

2 whole chicken breasts cut into mouth size cubed

2 tbsp. chili powder

3 tbsp. coconut oil

½ cup finely diced onion

½ cup finely diced celery

1 tsp. red chili flakes, more if you want it spicier

2 cloves of garlic finely chopped

1 tbsp. dried coriander

1 tbsp. dried cumin

1 large can of diced tomatoes

1 can of black beans

½ cup chopped fresh cilantro

Salt and pepper to taste

Melt 2 tbsp. of the coconut oil in a large skillet and add the chicken pieces. Add the chili powder and stir well. Take the chicken out of the skillet and set it aside. Melt 1 tbsp. of coconut oil into the skillet and add the vegetables and spices. Add the can of tomatoes, beans and the cooked chicken. Mix well. Add the fresh cilantro and stir. Simmer for an hour before serving. Garnish with some non-fat plain Greek yogurt, Daiya cheese, and additional fresh cilantro.

CURRIED CAULIFLOWER RISOTTO

1/2 head of cauliflower
3 tbsp. Earth Balance
2 minced cloves of garlic
1 finely chopped medium onion
1 cup fresh green beans chopped course
1/4 cup water
1/4 cup non-fat plain Greek yogurt
1/4 cup tomato paste
2 tbsp. cashew butter
1/2 tsp. curry powder
1/2 tsp. cinnamon
Dash of cayenne pepper
Dash of sea salt

Using a food processor, grate the cauliflower. Put the prepared cauliflower in a pot and pour the water over it. Boil for 3 minutes, drain and cool.

In a big frying pan melt the Earth Balance and then add the onion, garlic and beans. Gently sauté for about 5 minutes and then add all the rest of the ingredients. Add the cauliflower to the pan and gently mix into the rest of the ingredients.

SPINACH GNOCCHI

1 lb. fresh young spinach
3 egg yolks
1/4 lb. raw goat cheese
1/4 tsp fresh, finely grated nutmeg
Salt and pepper to taste
1/2 cup finely ground almond flour
Earth Balance or coconut oil for frying

Before you begin, you need to blanch the spinach. First, fill a large bowl with cold water and ice. Then, fill a large pot half way with water and bring to a full boil. Add the spinach and cook for 30 seconds, not any longer. Quickly remove the spinach, using a large slotted spoon or mesh sieve and put into the cold water. This will stop the cooking process. Remove the spinach from the cold water and squeeze out the water. Then place it on a tea towel and roll the towel, in order to get the last of the moisture out of the spinach.

Put the prepared spinach into a food processor along with the egg yolks and blend until the mixture is smooth. Next, add the goat cheese, nutmeg, salt and pepper. Continue mixing until well blended and smooth.

Remove ingredients from the food processor and put into a large mixing bowl. Add the almond flour and mix. Cover the bowl with plastic wrap and place in the fridge for 1 hour.

After the dough has rested for 1 hour, use a small spoon to scoop equal portions of mix and shape them into small ovals about the size of an olive. Place the ovals onto a cookie sheet, cover with plastic wrap and place back into the fridge for another 1/2 hour.

Boil a large pot of water and add the prepared gnocchi. Put the gnocchi into a frying pan that has had Earth Balance or coconut oil melted into it. Fry the gnocchi for just a moment, transfer to a plate and enjoy.

Tofu Skin Stir Fry

This is a great way to have an alternative to Asian noodles, without the noodles! Makes a great side for a veggie stir-fry. However, do not add any other ingredients with this cooking process, as it will moisten the tofu skins and change their consistency.

1 package fresh tofu skins (can be purchase at Asian markets)
1 tbsp. coconut oil
2 tbsp. Bragg's Amino Acids
1 tbsp. Xylitol
1 tbsp. chili oil
1 tbsp. sesame oil
1 tbsp. sesame seeds
3 green onions, chopped

Unfold the tofu skins and shred them by pulling apart into randomly shaped, thin pieces. In a large skillet melt the coconut oil. Add the shredded tofu skins and cook on medium, continuously tossing so that the skins become evenly browned.

In a large mixing bowl, add the rest of the ingredients and whisk well. Once the skins have browned, place them in the bowl with the mixture and continue tossing so they become evenly coated with the sauce. Then, return the whole mixture to the frying pan and continue fry for another 10 minutes. Keep tossing the mixture as you finish the cooking process.

Tofu Quinoa Fry

1 cup cooked quinoa
8 ounces extra firm non GMO organic tofu
2 tsp. olive oil
1 small red onion, finely chopped
1 medium red bell pepper, finely chopped

1/2 cup frozen peas

1 tbsp. minced garlic

Sea salt and pepper to taste

Cut tofu into cubes and set aside. In a frying pan, heat the oil and cook the onion and peppers for 8 minutes, then add the frozen peas and cook another 2 minutes. Add the prepared tofu and garlic and continue cooking for another 5 minutes. Add the quinoa that has been cooked and gently mix. Season to taste.

POACHED CHICKEN BREAST WITH GINGER

3 tsp. coconut oil

1 cup thinly sliced red onion

1 cup thinly sliced celery

1 tbsp. minced fresh ginger

1 tsp. curry powder

1 tsp. lime zest

1/4 tsp. red pepper flakes

2 cups vegetable or chicken stock (see recipes)

1 cup coconut milk

2 tbsp. fresh squeezed lime juice

2 cups green beans cut on an angle

4 chicken breast halves

1/4 cup chopped coriander leaves

Salt and pepper to taste

Serve over spaghetti squash (see recipe), quinoa, or sprouted brown rice.

In an oven safe, large pot or Dutch oven, melt the coconut oil and add the onion, celery, ginger, curry, lime zest and red pepper flakes. Sauté for approximately 3-5 minutes and then add the stock, coconut milk and lime juice. Simmer for 5 minutes. Add the chicken breast to the top of the mix and push down until submerged in the liquid. Simmer for another 20 minutes.

SOLE WITH ALMONDS

1 pound fillets of sole

Almond oil to coat the fillets

1/2 cup toasted, slivered almonds

Sea salt to taste

Preheat oven to 375 degrees. Clean the fish under cold running water. Pat dry with paper towels. Using the almond oil, lightly coat the fillets. Place them on a baking sheet lined with parchment paper. Sprinkle with the almonds and salt. Bake for 12 to 15 minutes (depending on the thickness of the fillets) and serve.

Fish Fillets with Cashews

1/2 cup cashews that is either raw or roasted

Herbs of choice (i.e. dill, tarragon, basil, lemon pepper, oregano)

Sea salt and pepper to taste

2 to 3 skinned white fish fillets (fish of your choice)

1/2 tsp. melted coconut oil

Preheat oven to 500 degrees. In a blender, grind the cashews and seasonings until fine.

Clean the fillets under cold water and pat a bit of the moisture away with paper towel. Do not dry them completely. Pour the melted oil over the fillets. Dredge the fillets in the ground mixture and place on a baking sheet that has been lined with parchment paper. Bake for 10 to 15 minutes, until they flake apart. Carefully remove and plate.

Bean and Quinoa Chili

1 cup rinsed and drained quinoa

2 cups water

1 tbsp. olive oil

1 large onion, diced

1 green bell pepper, seeded and diced

1 cup chopped celery

1/2 tsp. chili flakes

2 tomatoes, diced

1 cup carrots, diced

1 16 oz. can black beans, drained and rinsed

1 28 oz. can crushed tomatoes

1 tbsp. chili powder

1 tbsp. dried parsley

1 tbsp. dried oregano

2 tsp. ground cumin

1/2 tsp. black pepper

1/2 tsp. salt

4 green onions, chopped (reserve for plating)

Add quinoa to a saucepan, cover with water, simmer and cook until the liquid has been absorbed. Set aside. In a large pot, heat the oil and add the onion, bell pepper, celery and chili flakes. Sauté for about 5 minutes. Add the rest of the ingredients and cook on medium for 1/2 hour, remembering to stir intermittently. Before serving, add the quinoa and continue cooking on low for another 5 minutes. Plate and top with green onions.

AWESOME CHILI

1 tbsp. olive oil

1 onion, chopped

1/2 cup chopped green pepper

1/2 cup chopped red pepper

1/2 cup chopped orange pepper

1 lb. ground turkey

1, 16 oz. can navy beans, drained and rinsed

1, 28 oz. can shopped tomatoes

1 tbsp. chili powder

2 tsp. ground cumin

1 tsp. pepper

1 tsp. sea salt

2 cloves garlic, minced

1/2 cup water

1 tbsp. coconut oil or olive oil

In a large pot, heat the olive oil and add the onion and peppers. Cook for 5 minutes and then add the ground turkey. Continue cooking until cooked through. Add the remaining ingredients and bring to a boil. Reduce to a simmer and cook for approximately 1 hour. Alternatively you can place everything a crock pot, set on high and cook for 3–4 hours or low for 6-8 hours.

GINGER KALE

1 large bunch of kale

1 tbsp. olive oil

1 tbsp. coconut oil

2 cloves garlic, minced

1 medium onion, minced

1 tbsp. fresh ginger, minced

1 fresh lime, juiced

Pepper

Wash the kale and remove the thick ribbing. Cut the cleaned kale into strips. Using a steamer, steam the kale. In a large frying pan, heat the oil and add the rest of the ingredients, except the lime juice and pepper. Once the onion is translucent, add the kale and continue cooking until heated through. Pour on the lime juice and sprinkle with pepper. Toss and serve.

BOK CHOY FRY

2 tbsp. extra virgin olive oil

1 small onion, chopped

1/2 tsp. ginger, chopped

4 cloves garlic, chopped

1/2 tsp. sea salt

1/4 tsp. chili flakes

3 tbsp. vegetable stock

Juice of 2 lemons

1 medium sized batch of bok choy, chopped

In a wok, heat the olive oil and then add the ingredients, except for the broth, lemon juice and bok choy. Cook for 2 minutes and then add the last three ingredients.

STIR FRY KALE

1 large leek, cleaned and chopped thin

2 tbsp. extra virgin olive oil

1 can cooked beans (black-eyed peas, pinto, or chick pea) drained and rinsed

6 cups kale, washed and chopped (be sure to remove course veins and stem)

1/2 cup water

1 tsp. Bragg's Liquid Amino's

In a large frying pan or wok, add the olive oil and sauté leeks until tender. Add the beans and cook through. Next, add the kale and water. Cover and cook for approximately 15 minutes until the kale is tender. Sprinkle with Bragg's and serve.

LENTILS WITH SPINACH

3 cups spinach, chopped

2 cups canned lentils (drained and rinsed)

1 tbsp. fresh grated ginger

1/4 cup fresh squeezed lemon juice

Cayenne to taste

Sea salt to taste

In a skillet, add the spinach and lentils and cook for 5–10 minutes. Add the remaining ingredients and continue cooking for another 10 minutes.

RAW NORI

2 carrots cut in long strips

4 scallions cut in long strips

1 zucchini cut in long strips

1 cucumber cut in long strips

1 cup Alfalfa sprouts

1 tbsp. Bragg's Amino's

2 tbsp. fresh lemon juice

Nori sheets

Place all the prepared veggies in a large bowl and marinate in Bragg's and lemon juice for approximately 1 hour. Remove and dry on paper towels. Place the veggies on the Nori and top with sprouts. Roll up like sushi and enjoy.

Zucchini Casserole

1 cup cooked brown rice

2 cups zucchini, thinly sliced

1/2 cup chopped green onions

1/4 cup chopped fresh parsley

1/4 cup olive oil

2 beaten eggs

1/2 tsp. sea salt

1/4 tsp. garlic powder

1/2 tsp. oregano

Preheat oven to 350 degrees. Put all of the ingredients in a very large bowl and toss well. In a well-oiled casserole dish, put all of the mixed ingredients and bake for 1 hour.

Curried Chick Peas

1 shallot, chopped

1/2 cup vegetable stock

1 tbsp. curry powder

2 cups cooked chickpeas

1/2 cup coconut milk

1 tbsp. Italian parsley, chopped

Chili paste

In a saucepan, add the shallots, stock, curry powder and cook covered for 5 minutes on medium. Next, add the chickpeas and coconut milk. Leave the cover off and simmer for 20 minutes. Add the parsley and chili paste. Let rest for 5 minutes and serve.

Stir Fry Made Easy

1 tbsp. coconut oil

1 Leek, cleaned and chopped

10 Brussels sprouts, cleaned and sliced

4 cups Savoy cabbage, sliced

1 clove garlic, chopped

Pinch of chili flakes

Bragg's Liquid Amino's to taste

Finely cut chicken pieces that have been cooked

Using a wok, heat the oil, add leeks and cook briefly. Add the Brussels sprouts with a touch of water and cook briefly. Add the cabbage and another dash of water. Cover and cook for about a minute. Add the garlic, chili flakes and Bragg's. When almost done, add the cooked chicken to heat through and serve.

CITRUS FISH

First part of recipe:

2 white fish fillets

1 lime zest and juice

1/2 lemon zest and juice

1 tbsp. olive oil

1 small red chili

1 clove garlic, crushed

Sea salt and black pepper

Second part of recipe:

2 tsp. coconut oil

1 red onion, diced

2 cloves garlic, crushed

1/2 cabbage, sliced

Keep the fillets aside and add all the first part of the recipe ingredients in a large bowl and combine. Add the fillets and marinate for 1 hour in the fridge. Remove the fillets and cook in a skillet, browning on both sides. Don't overcook. Leave the fish to rest.

In a pan, heat the oil and add the onion and garlic and cook until soft, then add the cabbage and cook until soft but crunchy. Plate the cabbage and put the fish on top.

GARLIC SALMON AND TOMATOES

4 pieces of skinless salmon

4 medium tomatoes cut in half

1/2 tsp. paprika

2 tbsp. olive oil

3/4 tsp. salt

1/4 tsp. pepper

8 sprigs fresh thyme

4 cloves garlic, chopped

Turn on oven broiler. Put parchment paper on a cookie sheet and place the fish and tomatoes on top. Drizzle oil on salmon and tomatoes. Sprinkle paprika, thyme, salt, pepper and garlic on the salmon and tomato. Broil for approximately 10 minutes.

FANCY FISH

2 fish fillets

Juice of 2 limes

1 tsp. coconut oil

1 large stalk of lemongrass that has been ground

1 tsp. minced ginger

1/3 cup coconut milk

1 tbsp. cilantro

Put the lime juice in a shallow pan and add the fish to marinate for approximately 1 hour. Take the fish out of the marinade and sprinkle with the lemongrass, cilantro and ginger, making sure to get both sides. Use a glass baking dish that has been coated with coconut oil and place the fish in it. Pour the coconut milk over the fish and bake at 350 degrees for 35 minutes.

CHICKEN LETTUCE CUPS

1 medium onion, chopped

2 small baby bok choy cleaned and cut course

3 cloves garlic, chopped

1/2 lb. organic ground chicken or turkey

2 tsp. Bragg's Liquid Amino's

1/2 tsp. kelp powder (optional)

1/4 tsp. cayenne powder

1 egg (if tolerated)

1 tsp. coconut oil

1/4 head iceberg lettuce, cleaned and separated into cups

Stir fry the vegetable ingredients but keep crunchy. In another bowl, mix the chicken or turkey, Bragg's and cayenne. Add the egg, if tolerated. Then add the chicken or turkey mixture to the veggies and add the coconut oil. Cook on medium and continue stirring, keeping the chicken or turkey mixture broken up. Scoop the cooked mixture into the prepared lettuce cups.

CHICKEN STEW ITALIA

2 tbsp. coconut oil

2 stalks celery, cut into bite sized pieces

1 carrot, cut into bit sized pieces

1 small onion, chopped

Sea salt and pepper to taste

14 1/2 oz. can chopped tomatoes

14 oz. chicken stock

1/2 cup fresh basil leaves, torn

1 tbsp. tomato paste

1 bay leaf

1/2 tsp. dried thyme leaves

2 chicken breasts

15 oz. can kidney beans, drained and rinsed

In a large baking skillet, heat the oil and add the veggies. Cook until slightly tender. Season with salt and pepper. Stir in the tomatoes, tomato paste, stock, spices and chicken. Reduce heat to a simmer and cook for 1/2 hour. Remove the chicken breasts and cut into pieces that are bite size and let rest. Add the kidney beans and heat through. Place the chicken back into the skillet and bring to a simmer. Season to taste. Can be served with brown rice.

MEDITERRANEAN CHICKEN

4 chicken breasts

1/4 cup artichoke hearts chopped

7 oz. can roasted red peppers, chopped

2 tbsp. fresh basil, chopped

2 tbsp. pine nuts, roasted

2 tsp. lemon juice

1 tsp. olive oil

Salt and pepper to taste

3 tbsp. goat cheese (if tolerated)

Cut a slit in the chicken breast, without slicing through. Mix all the ingredients together and stuff the cavity with the mix. Place the rest of the mix on either side of the chicken, drizzle with olive oil and fry the prepared chicken breasts on medium heat, making sure to turn part way through cooking. Alternatively, you can place the prepared chicken breasts on a parchment paper lined baking sheet and bake at 350 degrees for 45 minutes, or until done.

STEWED MEATBALLS

1 lb. ground turkey

1 tsp. savory

1 tsp. basil

1 tsp. oregano

1/2 tsp. thyme

1/2 tsp. garlic powder

1 tsp. organic Herbamare seasoning salt

1 cup carrots, chopped

2 cups green beans, chopped

½ cup celery, chopped

2 cans diced tomatoes

2 cups red peppers, chopped

In a large bowl, mix the turkey and all seasonings. Form into balls and bake on a non-stick sheet in a 425 degree oven for 30 minutes. Steam all vegetables except tomatoes. Put all the ingredients in a large pot, along with the tomatoes and meatballs, and simmer until heated through.

SIMPLY ZUCCHINI PASTA

3 Zucchini's spiraled or sliced into ribbons with veggie peeler or spiralizer

15 cherry tomatoes, quartered

2 tbsp. coconut oil

2-3 cloves of garlic, minced

¼ cup pine nuts

Sautee garlic in coconut oil until slightly browned. Add in zucchini "noodles" and sauté for 3-4 minutes. Remove from heat. Top with cherry tomatoes and pine nuts.

ARTICHOKE, TOMATO AND CHICKEN VEGGIE BAKE

2 chicken breasts, cubed

1 medium zucchini quartered

2-3 cloves garlic, minced

1 tbsp. olive oil

1 can artichoke hearts in water, drained

2 stalks celery, chopped

1 cup carrots chopped

1 leek sliced fine

1 cup fresh parsley chopped

1 can organic BPA free diced tomatoes

Combine all ingredients into casserole dish and bake at 350° for 45-50 minutes or until chicken is thoroughly cooked.

LET THERE BE PIZZA!

1 coconut or flax pizza crust (see recipes in Baked Goods section)

Crushed tomato sauce

½ red pepper, chopped

½ zucchini, chopped

3-6 ounces roast chicken

2 tbsp. onion, diced

1-2 cups spinach, chopped

Top crust with all toppings placing spinach at the bottom. Cover with Daiya mozza cheese or crumbled goat cheese. Bake at 350° for 20 minutes. Enjoy!

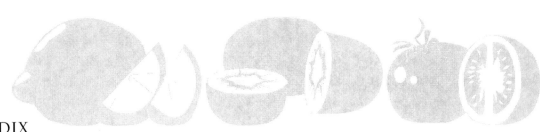

Appendix

Lab Testing

Diagnos-Techs

Comprehensive Digestive Stool Analysis

Stool Yeast Panel

19110 66th S, Bldg. G

Kent, WA 98032 USA

www.diagnostechs.com

Stero-Chrom Analytical

Food Allergy Testing

Serum Candida IgG/IgE Testing

7825 Edmonds Street

Burnaby, BC V3N 1B9 Canada

www.stero-chrom.com

Genova Diagnostics

Candida Immune Complexes

Anti-Candida Antibody

Candida Intensive Culture

Yeast Culture

Comprehensive Digestive Stool Analysis

63 Zillicoa Street

Asheville, NC 28801 USA

http://www.gdx.net/

SUPPLEMENTS:

DR COBI'S ONLINE STORE

All recommended supplements are available here
www.drcobi.com

AVICENNA

Pure Epsom salts
North Vancouver, BC Canada
http://www.avicennanatural.com/

DOUGLAS LABS

Douglas Laboratories | RIDC Location
112 Technology Drive
Pittsburgh, Pennsylvania 15108, U.S.A.
http://www.douglaslabs.com/index.cfm

INTEGRATIVE THERAPEUTICS

825 Challenger Drive
Green Bay, WI 54311 USA
http://www.integrativeinc.com/

METAGENICS

100 Avenida La Pata
San Clemente, CA 92673 USA
http://www.metagenics.com/

SEROYAL (GENESTRA)

490 Elgin Mills Road East
Richmond Hill, ON L4C 0L8 Canada
http://www.seroyal.com/

THORNE RESEARCH, INC.

P.O. Box 25
Dover, ID 83825 USA
http://www.thorne.com/

RECOMMENDED PROBIOTICS

- Seroyal HMF Replete
- Metagenics Ultra flora
- Douglas Labs 50 B and Multi 4000
- Klaire labs Therbiotic complete
- Transformation Enzymes Plantadophilus
- Innate Response: Food based probiotics
- Thorne Saccharomyces boulardii
- Bioimmersion Beta Glucan and probiotics maintenance
- Pharmax HCL intensive care and maintenance
- Dr. Ohira's probiotics
- Klaire ABX
- Natren—-health food store
- Custom Probiotics
- Bio-Kult
- Udo's Choice
- Jarrowdophillus
- Jigsaw
- Garden of Life
- Enzymatic Therapy

DRUGS FOR CANDIDA ELIMINATION

The following pharmaceutical medications are used in the conventional treatment of fungal overgrowths. Issues often return after treatment, when the underlying causes of the overgrowth have not been eliminated.

NYSTATIN

Nystatin was one of the first anti-fungal drugs developed and probably the most commonly used to treat intestinal yeast overgrowth. Nystatin kills yeast by binding to a specific compound, called ergosterol, found on yeast cell walls. Once bound, it causes the cell the leak, eventually causing its death. It is extremely safe due to the fact that hardly any of the drugs are absorbed from the intestinal tract. As a result, the only side-effects that may occur are mainly restricted to the digestive system and are usually mild. In addition, in rare cases patients may develop a rash as a result of an allergic reaction. Nystatin is available in a number of different forms including tablets, powder and liquid oral suspension. You can therefore choose the form that suits you best. The liquid and powder forms are probably superior to tablets because they don't need to be digested before they start to work and hence will kill yeast further up the digestive tract. The usual dosage of Nystatin ranges from 1 tablet or 1/8 of a teaspoon of powder 4 times a day to 8 tablets or 1 teaspoon 4 times a day.

AMPHOTERICIN B

This drug is similar to Nystatin as it is chemically related. As with Nystatin, it is not absorbed from the intestine in any significant amount so again is very safe. Amphotericin B may be effective in cases where Nystatin has failed. Amphotericin B binds to the ergosterol on the cell wall of yeasts damaging it and causing potassium to leak resulting in death of the cell.

DIFLUCAN (FLUCONAZOLE)

Diflucan belongs to a group of drugs called the 'azoles' and unlike the previous two drugs, Diflucan is absorbed by the intestines and is referred to as a systemic anti-fungal drug. Diflucan is a more modern drug than Nystatin and amphotericin. It was first used in Europe during the 1980's and licensed in the US in 1990. Many doctors and patients have found Diflucan (and other azoles) to be effective where Nystatin and amphotericin have failed. It has been found to be very safe considering its systemic action with few side-effects reported by patients. The dosage range is typically from 100 to 600mg a day with period of treatments ranging from a few weeks to many months, or in rare cases, indefinitely.

SPORANOX (ITRACONAZOLE)

Sporanox is one of the newest azole drugs and was licensed in the US in 1993. It would seem to be as similar in safety and effectiveness as Diflucan but may be a more successful treatment for certain species of Candida and other fungal infections whereas Diflucan may be more effective for other species.

NIZORAL (KETOCONAZOLE)

This drug was the first of the azole drugs to be developed but its use is limited due to the possibility of serious liver damage. As a result, patients must undergo regular liver enzyme tests during treatment to monitor and side effects on the liver. In cases that have failed to respond to any other anti-fungal agent, its use may be justified but otherwise it is probably best avoided.

LAMISIL (TERBINAFINE HCL)

This is the newest anti-fungal drug in routine use. It is a systemic drug but is unrelated to the other systemic 'azole' drugs. As a result, it is an effective treatment, as yeast has not yet had a chance to develop resistance to it. Lamisil has become more and more widely used since its introduction a few years ago and is set to become the systemic drug of choice, replacing Diflucan. As with most of the systemic drugs, there have been instances of adverse effects on the liver. Sporanox and Lamisil have also recently been linked with congestive heart failure.

HELPFUL CANDIDA INFORMATION WEBSITES

www.thecandidadiet.com

http://www.bodycleansing.org/candida-cleansing/

http://www.brendawatson.com/digestive-conditions/candida/

http://www.wholeapproach.com/

http://www.candidamd.com/treatment/index.html

http://functionalhealthtests.com/candida.html

http://candidaclinic.org/eliminating-systemic-candida/

http://www.becomehealthynow.com/article/conditionwomen/416/2/

http://www.modernherbalist.com/dieoff.html

http://drlwilson.com/articles/candida.htm

http://www.healingnaturallybybee.com/articles/intro2.php#s3

http://www.candidasupport.org/RESOURCES/comparing-candida-products/?gclid=COqujeu9nLlCFQjZQ-god1ncAIw

http://www.freecoconutrecipes.com/gluten_free_coconut_flour_recipes.htm

http://www.elanaspantry.com/ingredients/coconut-flour/

http://www.thecandidadiet.com/recipes.htm

http://www.candida-cure-recipes.com/natural-candida-cleanse.html

http://candidadietplan.com/candida-diet-recipes/candida-cleanse-recipes/

http://detoxinista.com/recipes/candida-cleansing-recipes/

Tawnies' testimonial is just one example of the thousands of Dr Cobi's patients that show how eliminating Candida can result in freedom from debilitating medical issues.

TAWNIES' STORY

"For as long as I can remember I've had digestive issues. I call them that because it's so much nicer than saying bloating, pain, weight-gain, diarrhea, constipation, and gas so shocking it could offend a skunk. I was brought up to not discuss those sorts of things. With all those secrets closely guarded I set out on my own (I couldn't possibly tell anyone — especially a doctor – how bad it really was) to try to figure out what was wrong with me. I tried elimination diets and cleanses, but my problems still didn't go away. I experimented with food combining and "clean eating" but my "digestive issues" were still front and centre. Eventually things got so bad that I couldn't ignore it and continue to pass it off as nothing more than a few little "digestive issues". I saw my doctor who referred me to a specialist, who I put off seeing for almost a year for fear of a colonoscopy. In June of 2009 my fear became reality and I had my first colonoscopy. The specialist told me that he'd found a large tumor in my sigmoid colon. It had been growing there for years, and due to its large size and difficult to reach location, it would have to be surgically removed. I was in shock. I couldn't understand how this could happen to me. After all, I'm a personal trainer and I live a clean, healthy life. I so foolishly believed that things like this only happen to people who eat fast food and don't exercise. The tumor, surrounding lymph nodes, and 20% of my colon were removed in August 2009 in an extremely invasive surgery called a colon resection. The tumor was cut out of my colon and the two healthy ends were reattached. I spent a week in the hospital hooked up to all sorts of machines, with drainage tubes and bags hanging off of me. I ate a steady diet of ice chips and lemon Jell-O and lost 13 pounds in less than a week. I experienced excruciating nerve pain in my arms and legs after surgery that lasted months. Yet I was one of the lucky ones! The tumor was in a pre-cancerous stage and it was caught before it had a chance to grow. The surgeon told me that these types of tumors grow quickly, and that if I had waited even just another 6 months my outcome would have been very different. I thought back to how long I'd put that initial appointment off with the specialist because I feared a colonoscopy. So foolish. Recovery was long and difficult, but I'd hoped to make a great come back and finally put all those nasty digestive issues behind me. The tumor was out and it had to be sunny skies from now on.

But that didn't happen. My digestive issues came back, only this time I had a short, angry colon to add to the mix. Here I go again trying to sugar coat it. What I should really say is that in addition to all my previous digestive symptoms, my short, angry colon resulted in 15 to 20 small bowel movements every day. I spent more time in the loo than anywhere else in my house! I told my doctor (because by this time I was liberated and could speak freely about all things "back door"). She called for more tests (3 CT scans and a partial colonoscopy to check for a bowel obstruction), all of which came up empty handed. My doctor suggested I try adding some fiber to my diet with Metamucil. Reluctantly I did, but it didn't help. Around this time my knees became incredibly swollen and painful, even from the smallest amount of activity. I saw a specialist who diagnosed me with advanced arthritis in one knee and moderate in the other. All 3 chambers of the knee were affected. I was 42 at the time, and the arthritis was so bad the x-ray technician kept asking me if I was sure I didn't sustain an injury. The specialist sat me down one day and told me that if I didn't stop running and all impact exercise, I'd be looking at a knee replacement within 2 years. I took the news gracefully, but inside I was screaming, "I'm a personal trainer with my own business! I can't just stop exercising!" I went home from that appointment so shattered and angry. It was definitely anger and rebellion that led me to put on my running shoes as soon as I got home and go for a run. In between tears and a lot of swear words; I managed to run the last 5km I would run for a very long time. I had no choice but to give in to my knee pain and stop running and all impact exercise. Just walking my kids to school became a painful ordeal. The swelling continued to get worse, even with no activity. My doctor tested me for lupus and thankfully it came back negative.

It didn't happen suddenly, but somehow over the next two years I became a shell of my former self. The passion I once had for my exercise classes was gone, my own fitness level declined rapidly, I lost confidence in myself, and I couldn't get motivated. I turned to food (and if I'm being completely honest, red wine) to numb my pain, and not surprisingly I gained weight. Oh and I still had all my "digestive issues" along for the ride! I was also dealing with terrible seasonal allergies, which my doctor was quick to prescribe a steroidal nasal spray and eye drops for. My life was falling apart right in front of my eyes. Weren't my 40's supposed to be the time of my life?

In early 2012 I decided to prepare myself for the possibility that I might not be able to continue in the fitness industry. I decided to go back to school and pursue Holistic Nutrition, while still teaching my group fitness classes. I have always been eager to learn about things I'm interested in, and nutrition was definitely one of those things. But I found it impossible to concentrate and therefore retain anything I read. My ability to stay focused was gone and my coursework progressed at a snail's pace. I sunk to even deeper levels of frustration and sadness. My muscles ached, my joints hurt, my allergies were awful, and my tummy was always in a state, and I couldn't exercise. I was a bloated, depressed, spaced-out, sorry excuse of a woman and I hid it from everyone.

In May 2012 I had my 3 year follow-up colonoscopy. I was almost certain they would find another tumor. I had all the same symptoms I had when they found the tumor the first time, and a whole bunch of new ones too. To my surprise the scope was clear. I was awake for the whole thing and I saw it all with my own eyes. It really was clear! I was relieved, but it still didn't explain why I continued to have all this pain and these horrible digestive issues.

In late May of 2012 I turned to Dr.Cobi. She was familiar with my history and somewhat familiar with my current concerns. I say somewhat because I hid them very well. After an initial questionnaire, she tested me for intestinal candida. The results were shocking. I had a big problem! I started treatment for intestinal candida and the 90 day candida detox diet immediately. The diet was a challenge. I didn't think I was going to make it, but I saw it through and completed the entire 90 days. There were a few rough spots in the first few weeks, but Dr.Cobi prepared me for them and supported me through them. In the weeks that followed, things got easier and I got into the routine of this new way of life. I even stopped keeping track of the days. My 90 day anniversary has come and gone and I'm totally converted. I say converted and not healed because I see how necessary it is for me to continue to eat this way. This is a way of life for me now, not just a quick fix. Here's why....my digestive issues are gone. I don't have any bloating, abdominal pain, constipation, diarrhea, or offensive gas. My stomach is finally happy! My allergies are gone. Gone! My muscle pain has improved dramatically. I've lost 10 pounds of body fat. I'm leaner and stronger than I've ever been. My knee pain is under control and I'm exercising again. My concentration has improved, my motivation is back, my energy levels are way up, my outlook on life is positive, my business is doing well, and I'm studying again. I feel fantastic! I have a renewed sense of myself and I'm filling up that empty shell with all the best parts of me that were missing for so long. But the most incredible part of this journey is that I'm running again. There aren't any marathons in my future, but being physically free to run when I want to run and not be in agony every step of the way is nothing short of a miracle to me. It's not so much about the act of running as it is about what it represents. Being able to run again symbolizes my freedom from my health issues. I'm moving forward, leaving the last 3 horrible years behind me and I couldn't have done it without Dr. Cobi. My candida monster is dead and I couldn't be happier or healthier. "

CPSIA information can be obtained at www.ICGtesting.com
Printed in the USA
LVOW09s0301280415

436356LV00005B/185/P